CONTENT

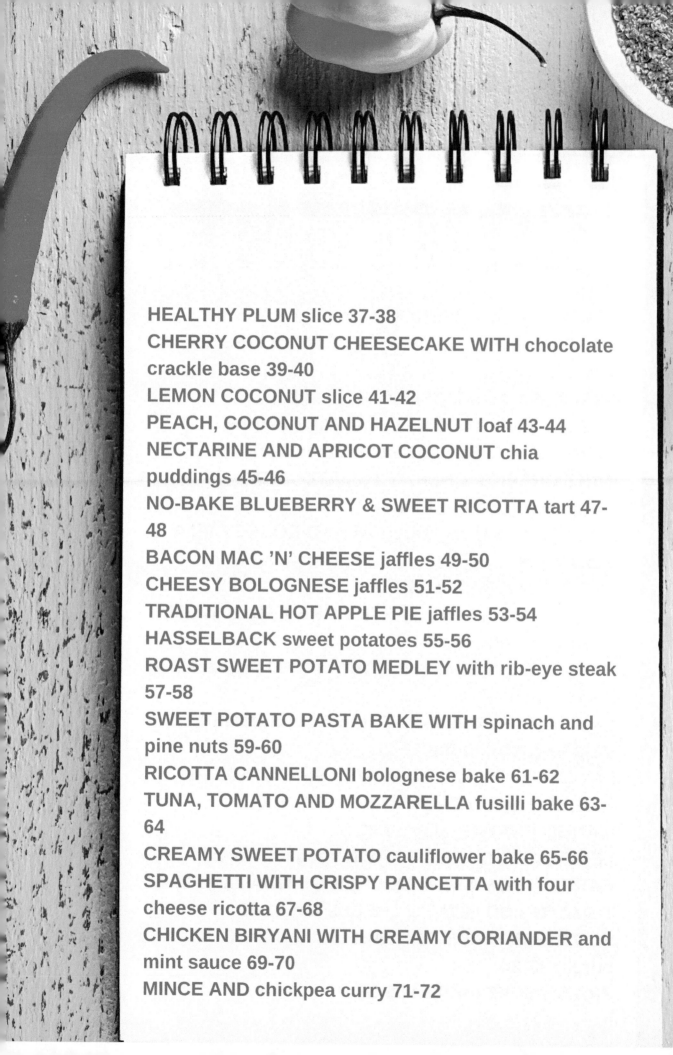

HEALTHY PLUM slice 37-38

CHERRY COCONUT CHEESECAKE WITH chocolate crackle base 39-40

LEMON COCONUT slice 41-42

PEACH, COCONUT AND HAZELNUT loaf 43-44

NECTARINE AND APRICOT COCONUT chia puddings 45-46

NO-BAKE BLUEBERRY & SWEET RICOTTA tart 47-48

BACON MAC 'N' CHEESE jaffles 49-50

CHEESY BOLOGNESE jaffles 51-52

TRADITIONAL HOT APPLE PIE jaffles 53-54

HASSELBACK sweet potatoes 55-56

ROAST SWEET POTATO MEDLEY with rib-eye steak 57-58

SWEET POTATO PASTA BAKE WITH spinach and pine nuts 59-60

RICOTTA CANNELLONI bolognese bake 61-62

TUNA, TOMATO AND MOZZARELLA fusilli bake 63-64

CREAMY SWEET POTATO cauliflower bake 65-66

SPAGHETTI WITH CRISPY PANCETTA with four cheese ricotta 67-68

CHICKEN BIRYANI WITH CREAMY CORIANDER and mint sauce 69-70

MINCE AND chickpea curry 71-72

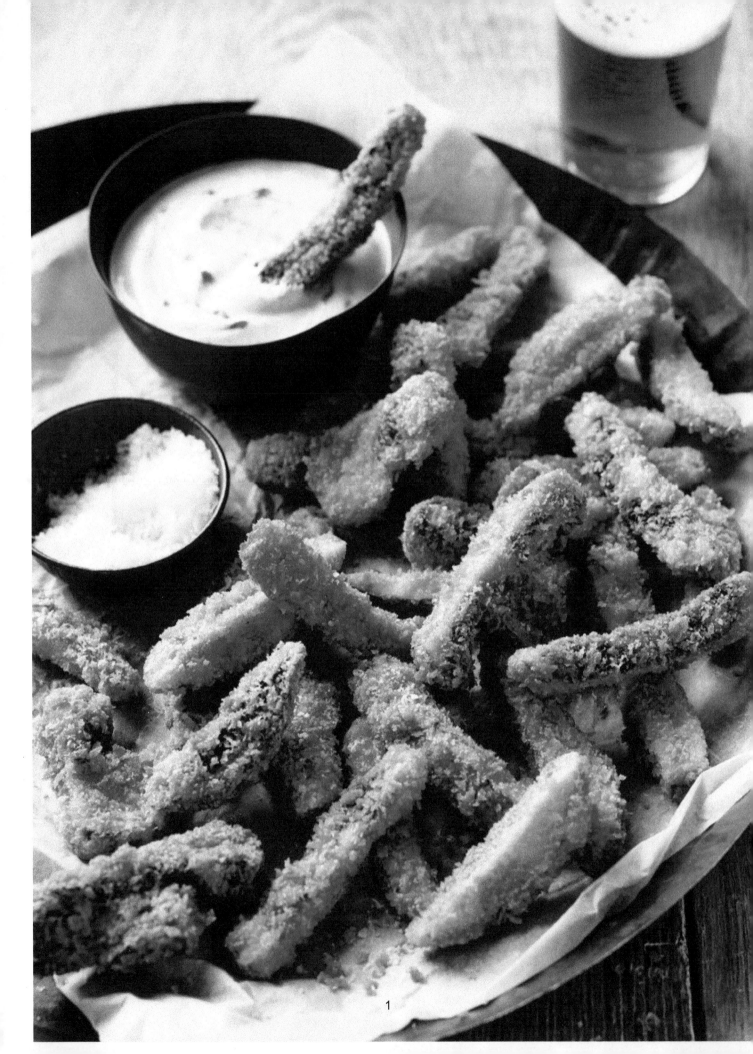

PORTABELLA MUSHROOM *fries*

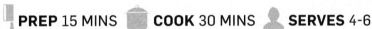 **PREP** 15 MINS **COOK** 30 MINS 👤 **SERVES** 4-6

INGREDIENTS

FRIES

Vegetable oil, for deep-frying

100g (⅔ cup) plain flour

3 eggs, lighly beaten

2 cups panko breadcrumbs

250g Portabella Mushrooms, stalks trimmed, cut into thin fries

Salt and pepper, to season

HARISSA YOGHURT

2 tsp harissa

1 cup Greek-style yoghurt

METHOD

FRIES

1. Heat enough oil in a large saucepan to come one-third up the sides to 170°C.

2. Meanwhile, place the flour, eggs and breadcrumbs into 3 separate wide, shallow bowls.

3. Season the flour well with salt and pepper. Dust the mushroom fries in the flour, shaking off any excess, dip into the egg, then coat well in the breadcrumbs.

4. In batches, deep-fry the fries for 5 minutes or until golden and cooked. Drain well on paper towel and season with salt.

HARISSA YOGHURT

1. Mix harissa together with yoghurt. Serve with fries.

TIP AND HINTS:

You can also use large flat white mushrooms, if you prefer

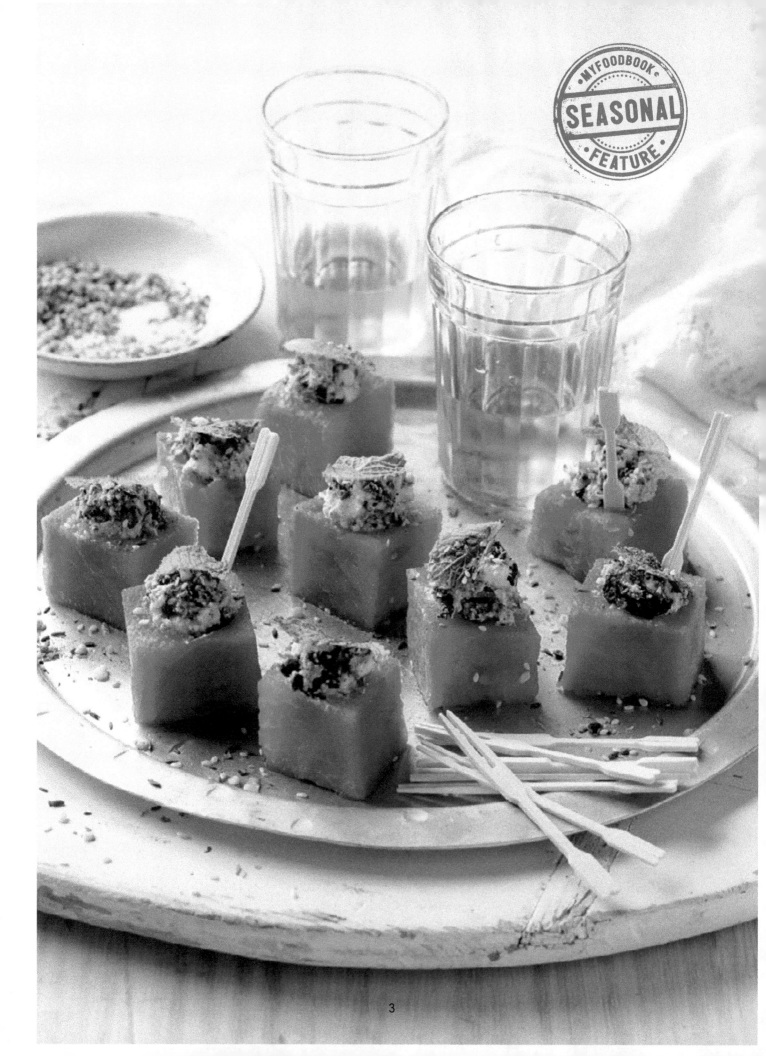

WATERMELON CUBES WITH FETA, OLIVES
and mint

 PREP 20 MINS   👤 **MAKES** 12

INGREDIENTS

½ small (about 2kg) piece seedless watermelon, chilled

100g Persian or marinated feta, drained

1 tbs finely chopped mint leaves, plus 12 small mint leaves, to serve

6 pitted Kalamata olives, finely chopped

Dukkah, to serve

METHOD

1. Trim watermelon and cut flesh into 12 x 3cm square cubes. Using a melon baller (or small knife), scoop a small well out of each watermelon cube, ensuring that you keep the watermelon sides intact.

2. Beat feta in a small bowl until smooth. Stir in mint and olives. Spoon mixture into watermelon cubes. Top each with a small mint leaf. Place onto a serving tray, sprinkle with dukkah and serve.

TIPS & HINTS:

Excellent for easy entertaining, serve these with cool drinks. Toss leftover watermelon through a fruit salad or blend it for an iced drink.

Dukkah is a delicious mixture of ground seeds, spices and nuts. It's available from some greengrocers and most supermarkets.

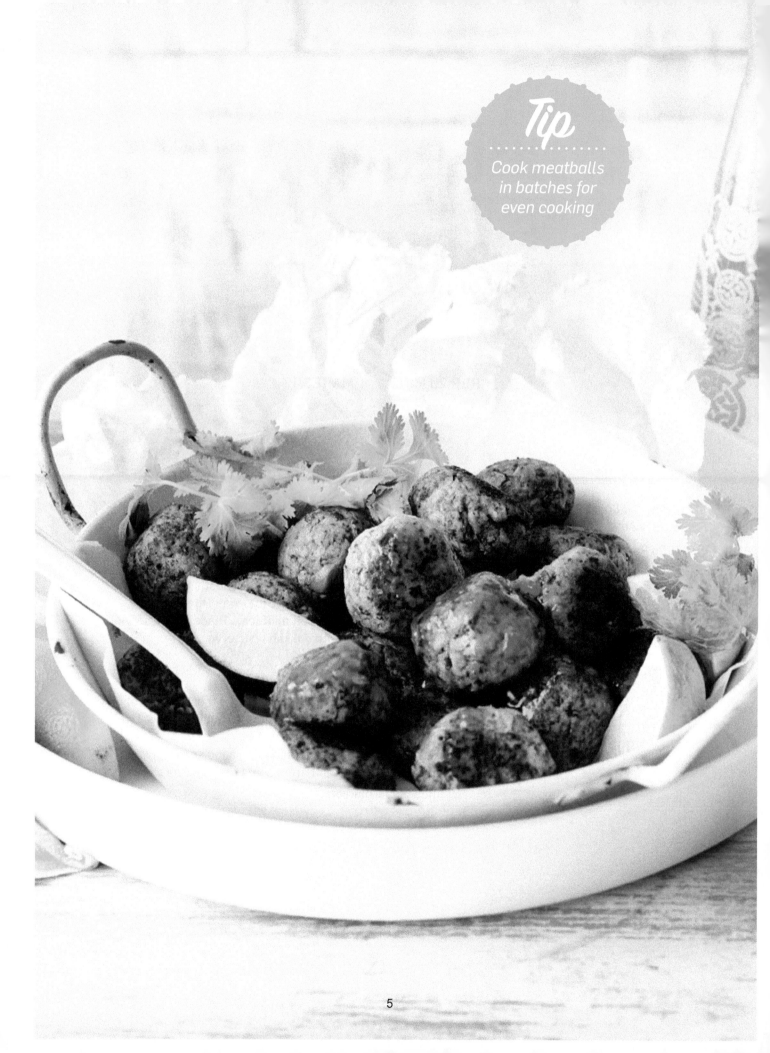

Tip

Cook meatballs
in batches for
even cooking

THAI PORK AND MUSHROOM
meatballs

 COOK 30 MINS **SERVES** 4

INGREDIENTS

400g button, cup or flat mushrooms

3 green onions, roughly chopped

3 tbs vegetable oil

2 tbs coriander paste or lightly dried coriander

400g pork mince

2 tbs red curry paste

1 egg

1 cup fresh breadcrumbs

Vegetable oil, for cooking

Iceberg lettuce, sweet chilli sauce and lime wedges, to serve

METHOD

1. Finely chop mushrooms by hand or alternatively, pulse in a food processor. Add chopped green onions to mushroom mixture.

2. Heat 1 tbs oil in a large non-stick frying pan over high heat. Add mushroom mixture and cook, stirring often, for 8 minutes or until all moisture has evaporated. Set aside to cool for 10 minutes. Drain any excess moisture and transfer mushrooms to a bowl. Wipe pan clean.

3. Add coriander paste to the mushrooms with the mince, curry paste, egg and breadcrumbs, mix until well combined.

4. Shape into balls with damp hands. Place onto a tray, cover and refrigerate 1 hour if time permits (this helps hold meatballs together when cooking).

5. Heat remaining oil in a large non-stick frying pan over medium heat. Cook meatballs, in batches for 8-10 min, shaking pan often or until just cooked through. Serve with lettuce leaves, sweet chilli sauce and lime wedges.

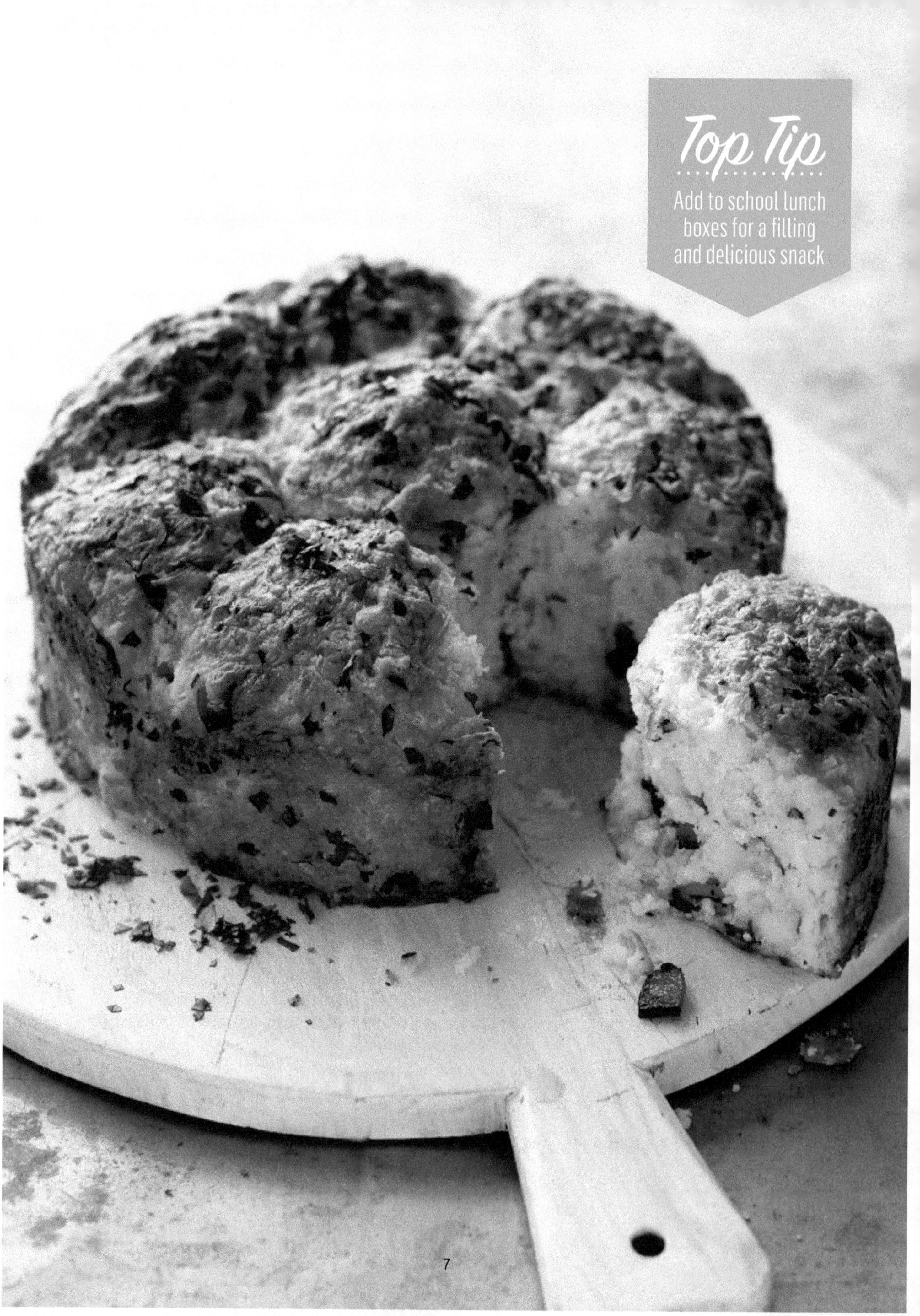

Top Tip

Add to school lunch boxes for a filling and delicious snack

CHEESE AND BACON PULL-APART
loaf

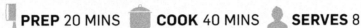 **PREP** 20 MINS **COOK** 40 MINS **SERVES** 8

INGREDIENTS

150g (6 rashers) rindless streaky bacon, chopped

450g (3 cups) self-raising flour

90g cold Fairy Cooking Margarine, chopped into 1 cm pieces

125g (1¼ cups) grated mozzarella

150g (1¼ cups) grated vintage cheddar

2 eggs

180ml (¾ cups) milk

½ cup fresh parsley, chopped

METHOD

1. Preheat oven to 180°C (fan forced). Grease and line the base of a 20cm round tin with baking paper. Grease the sides of the tin.

2. Cook the bacon in a small frying pan over high heat for 2-3 minutes or until golden brown.

3. Put the flour in a large bowl. Add the Fairy Cooking Margarine and use your fingers to rub the margarine into the flour until sandy. Add 1 cup of mozzarella, 1 cup of cheddar and the bacon. Use a butter knife to mix until combined.

4. Beat the eggs and milk together. Add to the flour mixture and use a butter knife to stir together to form a dough. Turn out onto a floured kitchen bench and gently knead together. Divide into 8 balls.

5. Put the remaining mozzarella, remaining cheddar and parsley in a small bowl and mix to combine. Roll each of the balls of dough into the cheese mixture. Place into the prepared tin.

6. Bake for 35 minutes, or until the bread is golden brown and cooked.

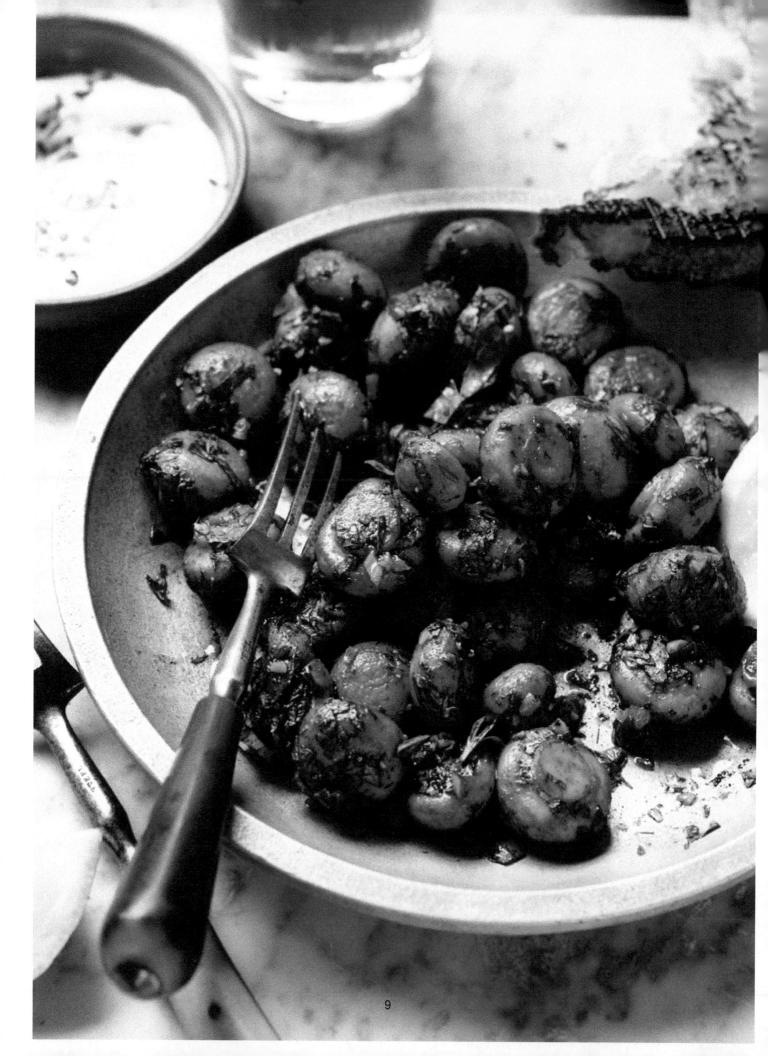

TAPAS STYLE GARLIC *mushrooms*

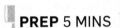 **PREP** 5 MINS 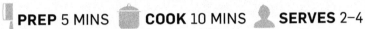 **COOK** 10 MINS 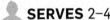 **SERVES** 2–4

INGREDIENTS

2 tbsp olive oil

250g button mushrooms, cleaned

4 garlic cloves, finely chopped

2 tsp smoked paprika

2 tbsp finely chopped parsley

Salt and pepper, to season

Aioli and lemon wedges, to serve

METHOD

1. Heat the oil in a large frying pan over medium-high heat. Cook the mushrooms for 5 minutes, tossing the pan regularly. Add the garlic, smoked paprika, salt and pepper and cook for a further 1-2 minutes or until golden, tossing the pan regularly. Toss through the parsley to combine

2. Serve the mushrooms with aioli and lemon wedges

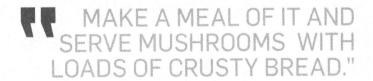

" MAKE A MEAL OF IT AND SERVE MUSHROOMS WITH LOADS OF CRUSTY BREAD."

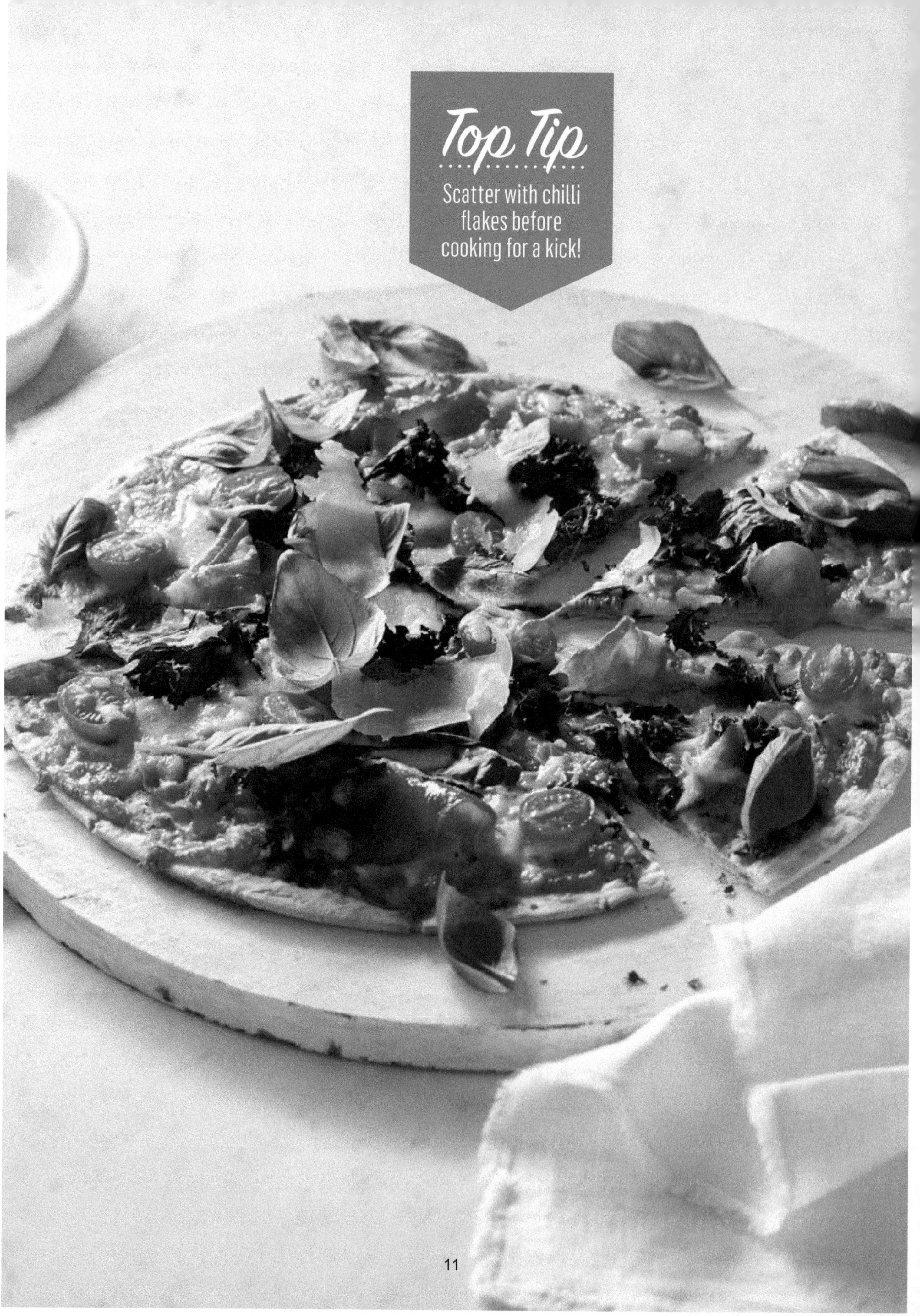

BABY GREENS, CHERRY TOMATO AND PROSCIUTTO

pizza

 PREP 5 MINS **COOK** 15 MINS **MAKES** 1 LARGE

INGREDIENTS

1 large pizza base

3 tbsp tomato passata

5 slices prosciutto

½ cup mixed kale and spinach leaves

250g Perfect Italiano Perfect Pizza

½ cup cherry tomatoes, halved

8-10 basil leaves

Shaved Perfect Italiano Parmesan, to serve

METHOD

1. Preheat oven to 250°C.

2. Spread the pizza base with tomato passata. Arrange the prosciutto, cherry tomatoes, kale and spinach on top of pizza. Scatter with Perfect Italiano Perfect Pizza to evenly cover base.

3. Place the pizza in the oven for 10–15 minutes or until the cheese is melted and base is crispy. Remove from the oven, scatter with Perfect Italiano Shaved Parmesan and basil and serve immediately.

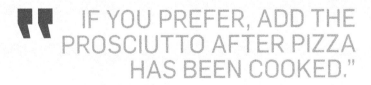

" IF YOU PREFER, ADD THE PROSCIUTTO AFTER PIZZA HAS BEEN COOKED."

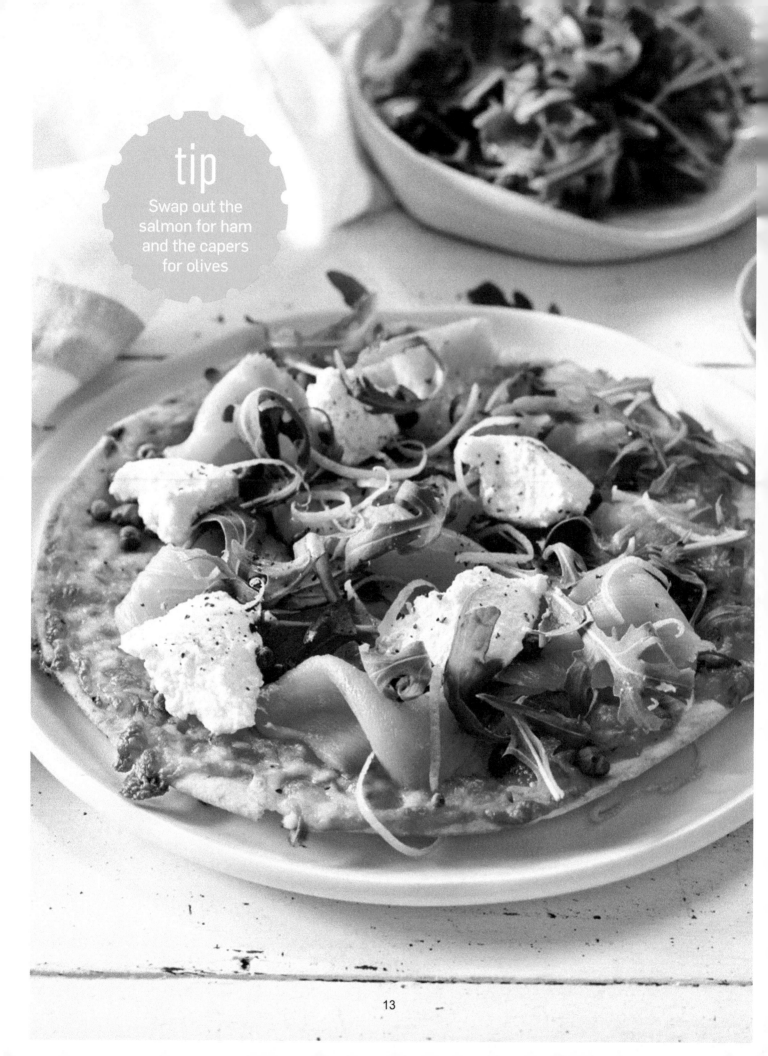

tip

Swap out the
salmon for ham
and the capers
for olives

SMOKED SALMON, RICOTTA AND ROCKET PITA
pizza

 PREP 5 MINS   **COOK** 15 MINS   **MAKES** 1 LARGE

INGREDIENTS

1 medium pitta bread

2 tbsp tomato passata

100g Tassal Smoked Salmon

250g Perfect Italiano Perfect Pizza

1 tbsp Always Fresh Capers, drained

⅓ cup baby rocket leaves, to serve

⅓ cup Perfect Italiano Ricotta

Zest of half a lemon

METHOD

1. Preheat oven to 250°C.

2. Spread the pitta with tomato passata. Scatter with Perfect Italiano Perfect Pizza to evenly cover base.

3. Place the pizza in the oven for 10-15 minutes or until the cheese is melted and base is crispy. Remove from the oven, lay over slices of smoked salmon, sprinkle over capers, and rocket leaves. Dollop on spoonfuls of Perfect Italiano Ricotta, sprinkle over lemon zest and season with salt and pepper. Serve immediately.

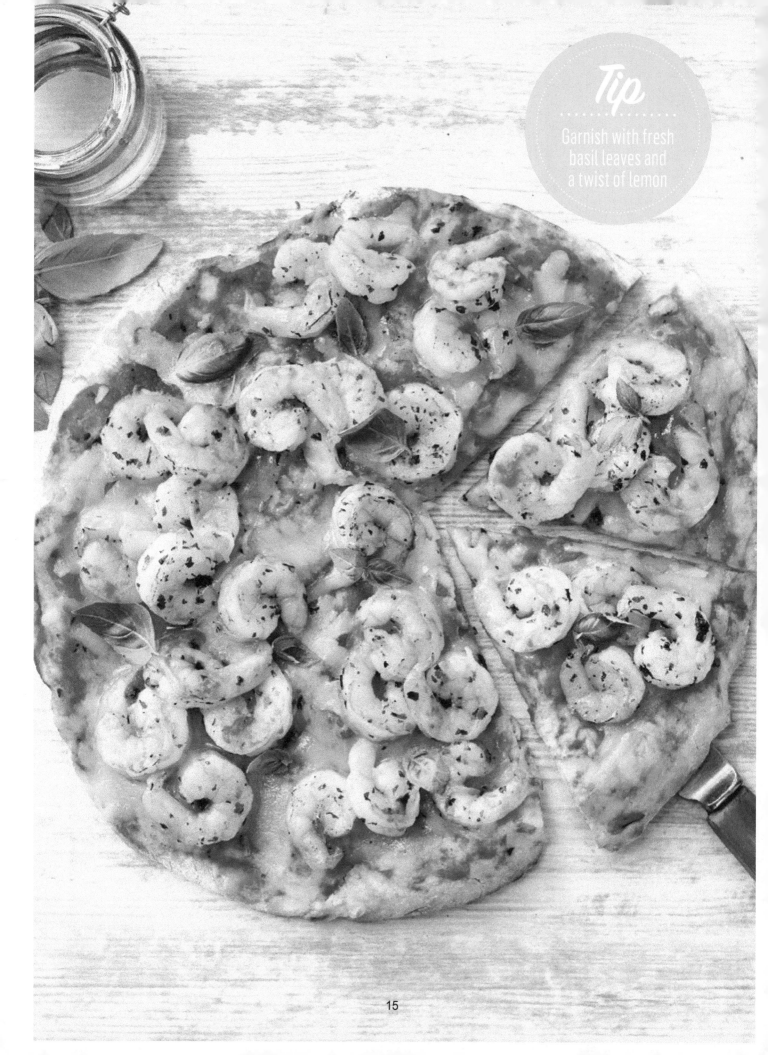

EASY PRAWN
Pizza

 PREP 15 MINS   **COOK** 10 MINS **SERVES** 4

INGREDIENTS

PIZZA

1 x any of the De Costi Prawn Range

½ pizza tomato paste

2 prepared thin pizza bases

1 cup pizza cheese

TO GARNISH

Fresh basil leaves

METHOD

PIZZA

1. Pre-heat oven 200°C.
2. Spread the tomato paste over the base and sprinkle the cheese evenly over the pizza base.
3. Mix De Costi Prawns in a bowl and divide evenly over the pizza bases.
4. Bake the pizzas for 5 minutes or until cheese is bubbly and beginning to look golden.

TO GARNISH

1. Slice pizza into wedges and garnish with basil leaves. Serve immediately.

TIPS & HINTS:

Spice up your pizza with a little chipotle mayonnaise for a delicious difference.

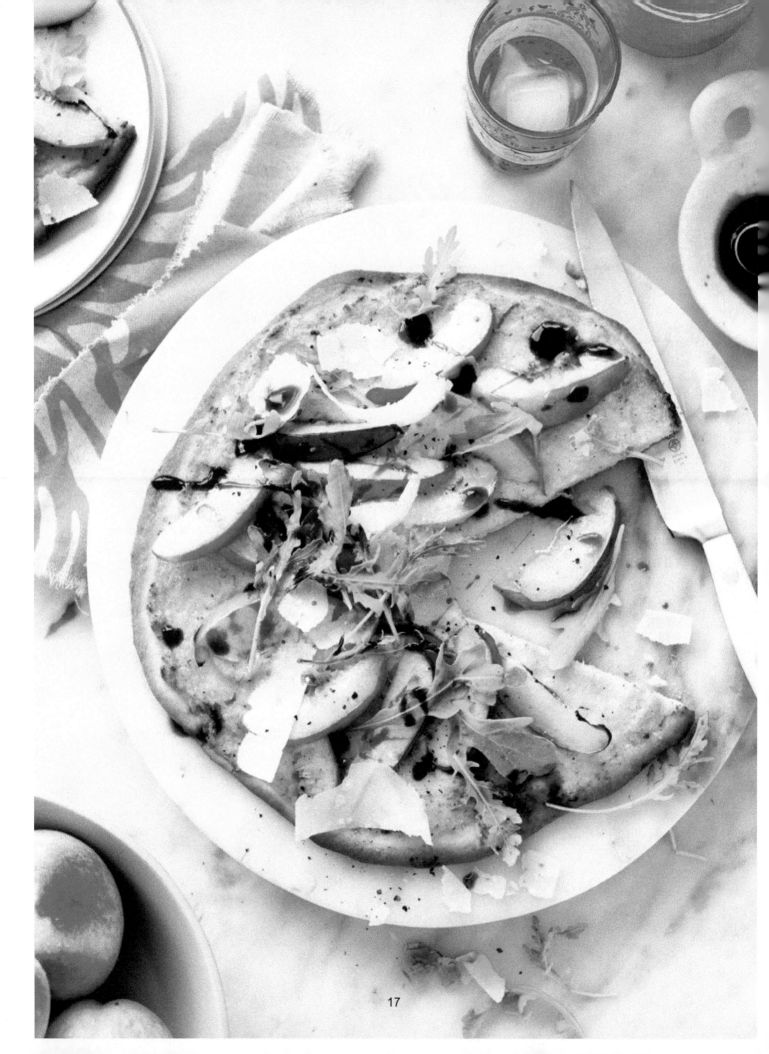

YELLOW NECTARINE, ARTICHOKE AND ROCKET

pizza

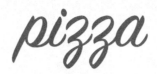 **PREP** 25 MINS + PROVING TIME   **COOK** 15 MINS   **SERVES** 4

INGREDIENTS

¾ cup hot water

2 teaspoons instant yeast

1 teaspoon caster sugar

2 cups pizza flour

1 teaspoon sea salt flakes

⅓ cup olive oil

280g jar whole artichoke hearts, drained

½ cup finely grated parmesan

3 firm yellow nectarines, cut into thin wedges (approx. 180g each)

Shaved parmesan, to serve

20g baby rocket

⅓ cup balsamic glaze

METHOD

1. Whisk water, yeast and sugar in a jug and set aside for 10 minutes or until mixture is frothy. Place flour and salt into a large bowl. Add yeast mixture and 1 tablespoon oil. Stir until well combined and a soft dough forms. Turn onto a lightly floured surface and knead for 5 minutes or until a smooth dough forms. Place into an oiled bowl and set aside in a warm place for 30 minutes or until well risen.

2. Meanwhile, place artichoke, remaining ¼ cup oil, parmesan, salt and white pepper into a small food processor and pulse until a thick paste forms.

3. Preheat oven to 240°C. Grease 2 large baking trays. Punch down dough and divide in half. Roll one piece of dough on a lightly floured surface until approximately 25cm round. Place on prepared tray. Repeat with remaining dough.

4. Spread artichoke paste onto pizzas. Top with nectarine wedges and bake for 10-15 minutes or until pizza is golden and crisp. Top with shaved parmesan and rocket. Drizzle with balsamic glaze and serve immediately.

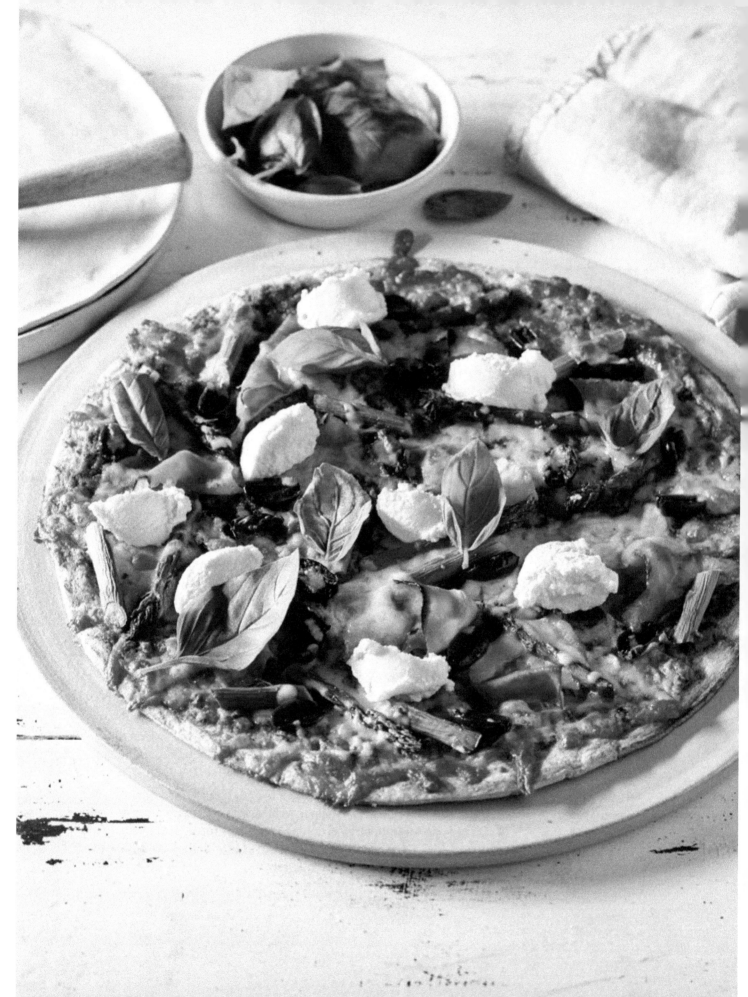

HAM, OLIVE, ASPARAGUS AND RICOTTA
pizza

PREP 5MINS   **COOK** 15 MINS   **MAKES** 1 LARGE

INGREDIENTS

1 large pizza base

3 tbsp basil pesto

100g ham, torn into large pieces

½ bunch asparagus, trimmed and chopped into thirds

½ cup pitted kalamata olives

250g Perfect Italiano Perfect Pizza

⅓ cup Perfect Italiano Ricotta

6-8 basil leaves, to serve

METHOD

1. Preheat oven to 250°C.

2. Spread the pizza base with pesto. Arrange the ham, asparagus and olives on top of the pizza. Scatter with Perfect Italiano Perfect Pizza to evenly cover base.

3. Place the pizza in the oven for 10-15 minutes or until the cheese is melted and base is crispy. Remove from the oven and spoon over dollops of Perfect Italiano Ricotta and sprinkle over fresh basil leaves. Serve immediately.

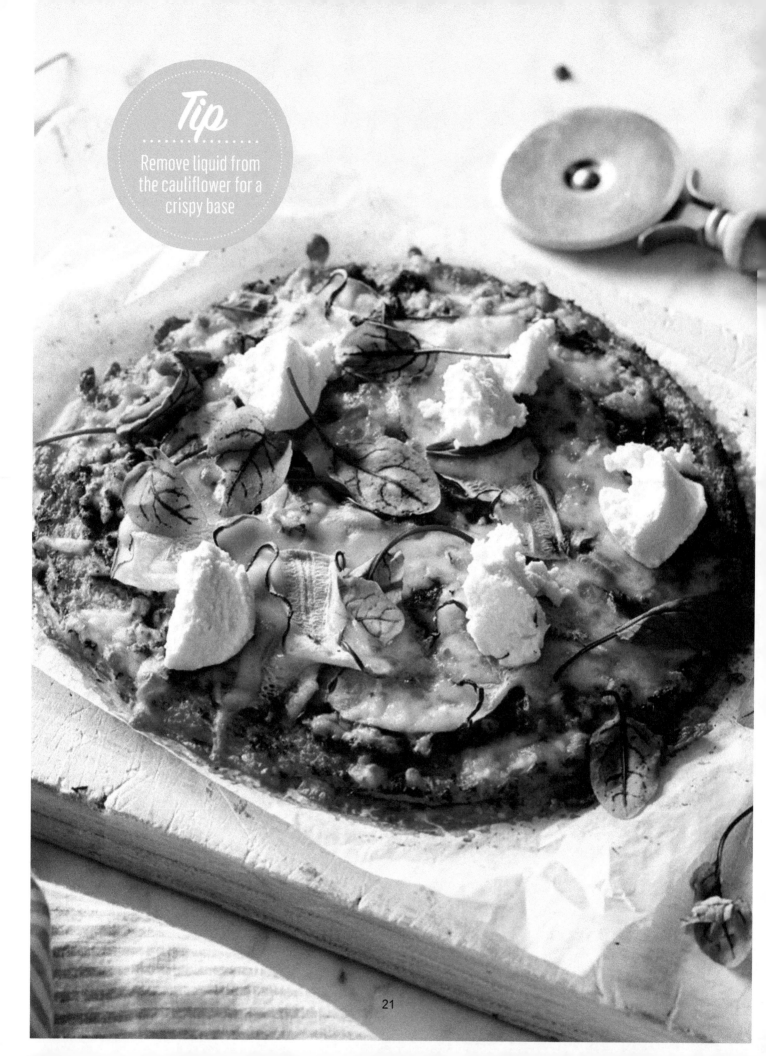

CAULIFLOWER PIZZA WITH PESTO, SUMMER VEGGIES

and ricotta

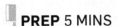 **PREP** 5 MINS   **COOK** 15 MINS **MAKES** 1 LARGE

INGREDIENTS

1 large cauliflower, florets removed and blitzed into rice (around 2 cups)

1 egg, lightly whisked

2 tbsp basil pesto and cashew dip

1 zucchini, trimmed and sliced into ribbons using a peeler

25g Perfect Italiano Grated Parmesan

250g Perfect Italiano Perfect Pizza

⅓ cup Perfect Italiano Ricotta

5-6 sorrel, to serve

METHOD

1. Preheat oven to 220°C.

2. To make the cauliflower crust, place cauliflower rice into a microwave safe bowl and microwave for 6-8 minutes or until very tender. Drain through a fine sieve and press down firmly with a spoon to remove all excess liquid (alternatively, wrap up in a clean chux and squeeze out all the excess liquid). Place cauliflower into a medium bowl and mix well with egg, parmesan and season with salt and pepper.

3. Line a baking tray with baking paper, and press cauliflower mixture firmly onto the tray forming a circle around 30cm. Place into the oven and bake for 20 minutes or until firm and golden. Remove from oven and allow to cool for 5 minutes.

4. Spread cauliflower base with basil pesto and cashew dip. Arrange the zucchini on top of pizza. Scatter with Perfect Italiano Perfect Pizza to evenly cover base.

5. Place the pizza in the oven for 10 minutes or until the cheese is melted and base is crispy. Remove from the oven, dollop spoonfuls of Perfect Italiano Ricotta on top of pizza, sprinkle over sorrel leaves and serve immediately.

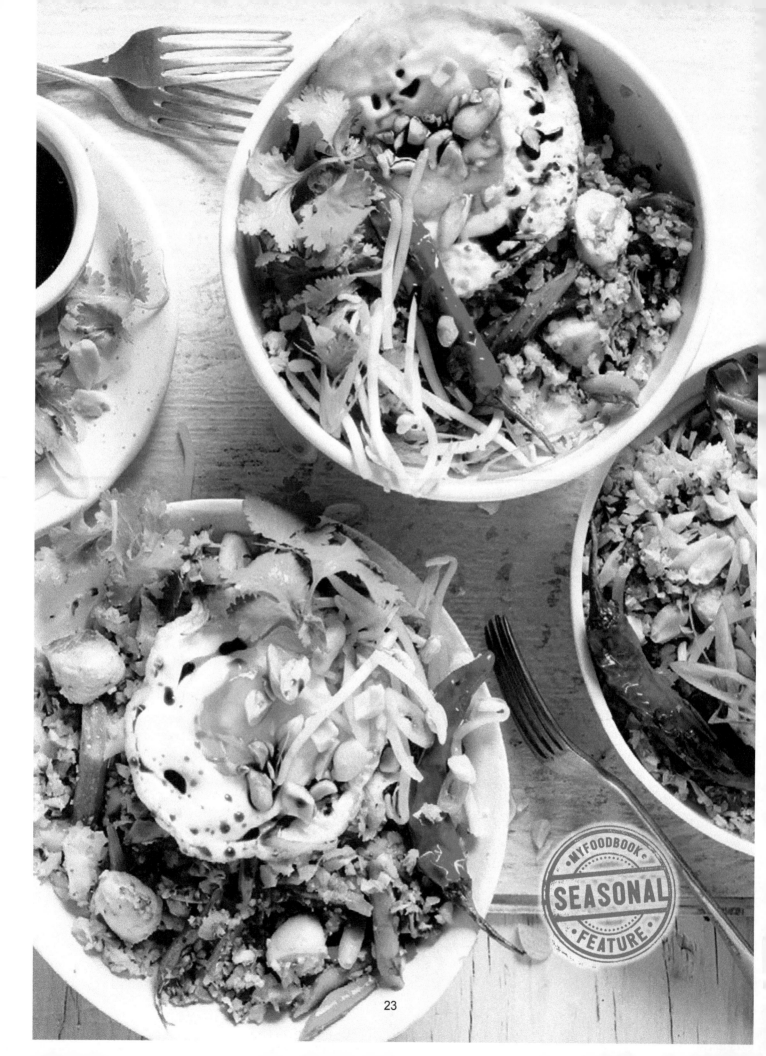

BROCCOLINI & CAULIFLOWER FRIED 'RICE' & CHICKEN
bowls

 PREP 30 MINS **COOK** 20 MINS **SERVES** 4

INGREDIENTS

2 bunches broccolini, roughly chopped

600g cauliflower florets (about ½ large cauliflower)

¼ cup peanut oil

4 free-range eggs, at room temperature

4 long red chillies (leave whole)

400g chicken tenderloins, trimmed and cut into 2cm pieces

3 green onions (shallots), trimmed and thinly sliced, plus extra to serve

2 garlic cloves, finely chopped

150g green beans, cut into 3cm lengths

2 tbs kecap manis, plus extra to serve

1 cup trimmed bean sprouts

½ cup coriander leaves

chopped roasted peanuts, to serve

METHOD

1. Preheat oven to 100°C fan-forced. Using a food processor, pulse broccolini and cauliflower in batches until it resembles rice. Set aside.

2. Heat 1 tbs oil in a wok over high heat. Fry eggs one a time until crisp at the edges and whites are set. Transfer to a tray and keep warm in the oven. Add another 1 tbs oil to wok and fry chillies for 1-2 minutes until crisp. Transfer to the tray and keep warm in the oven.

3. Heat remaining 1 tbs oil in the wok over high heat. Add chicken and stir-fry for 2-3 minutes until white and sealed. Transfer to a plate. Add green onions, garlic and beans to wok and stir-fry for 1 minute. Toss through broccolini and cauliflower 'rice' and stir-fry for 2-3 minutes until just tender. Drizzle with kecap manis and toss to combine.

4. Spoon into serving bowls. Top each with an egg and a fried chilli. Sprinkle with bean sprouts, coriander and extra green onions. Serve with chopped roasted peanuts and extra kecap manis.

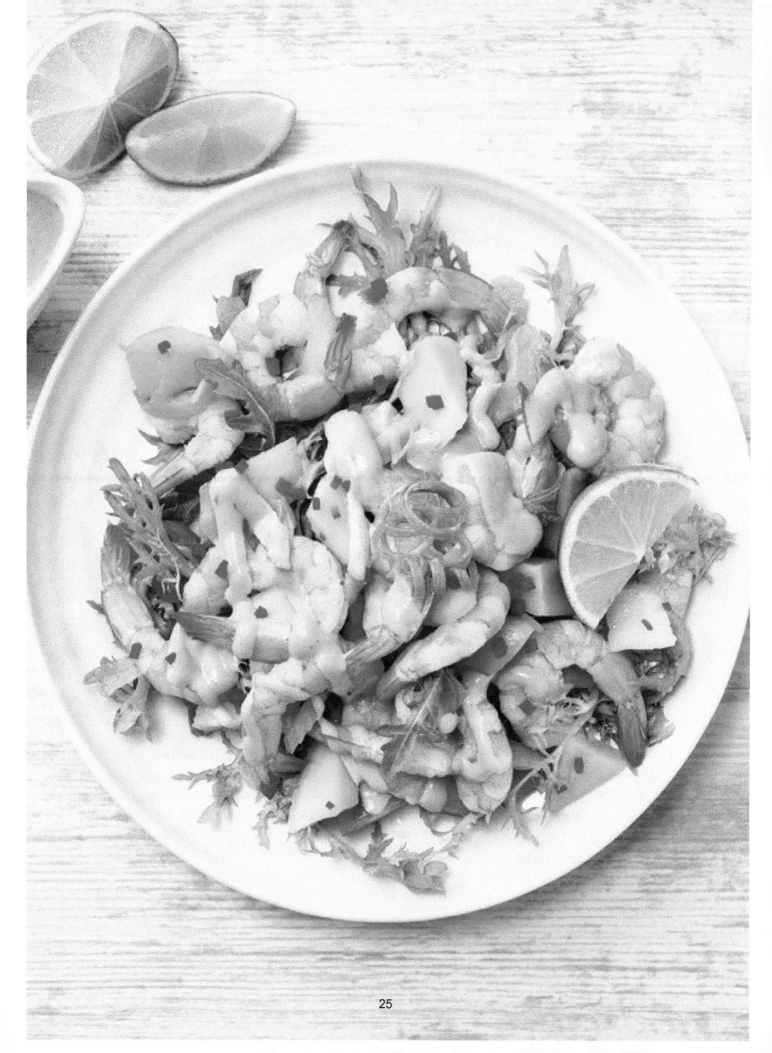

MANGO PRAWN
salad

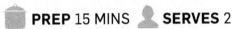 **PREP** 15 MINS **SERVES** 2

INGREDIENTS

1 x 260g DeCosti Cooked Prawns
with Cocktail Sauce

1 fresh Ripe Mango, diced

½ Red Capsicum, finely diced

50g Rocket Leaves

GARNISH

Lime Wedge

METHOD

1. Add the diced Mango, DeCosti cooked prawns to a large bowl along with the diced capsicum and rocket leaves.

2. Open the dressing pack and squeeze in half the dressing. Gently toss the dressing through the prawn and mango mixture.

3. Serve the Mango Prawn salad garnish with a wedge of lime and a little extra dressing.

NOTES:

Salad maybe prepared ahead of time and dressed just prior to serving.

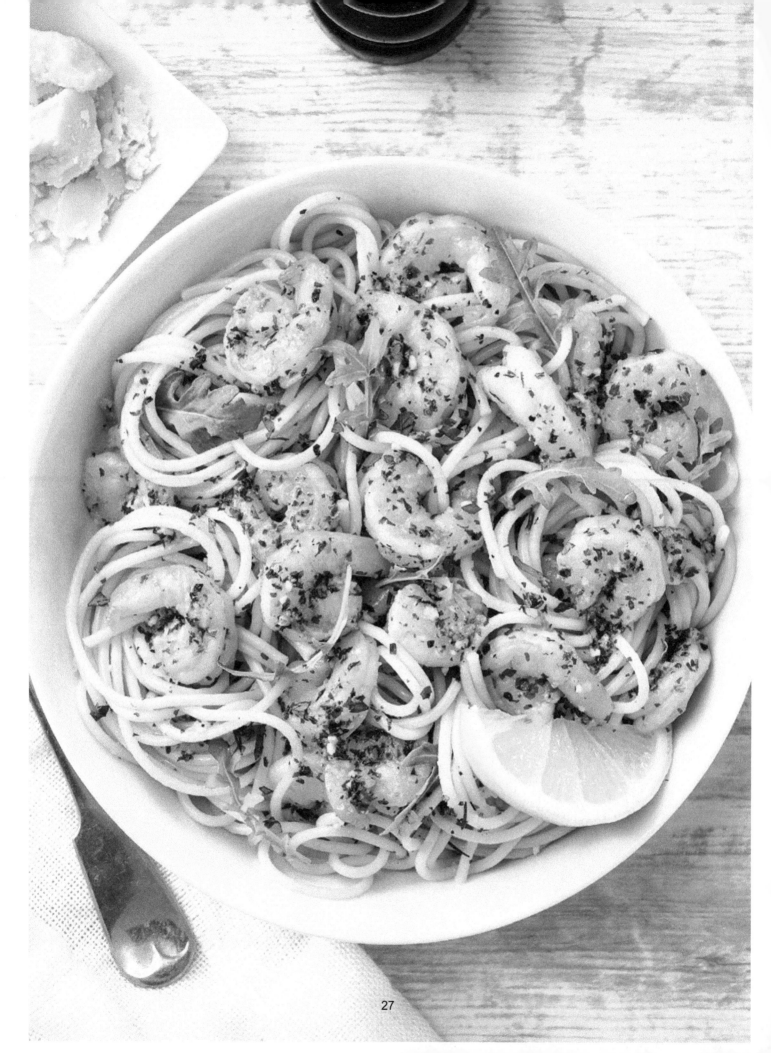

LEMON AND GARLIC PRAWN
spaghetti

 PREP 7-10 MINS **COOK** 6 MINS 👤 **MAKES** 4

INGREDIENTS

1 x 280g De Costi Prawns with Lemon & Garlic butter

½ packet of spaghetti, cooked and drained

1 tbsp of oil

Baby rocket, to serve

Fresh basil and sliced lemon, to serve

Salt and pepper, to season

METHOD

1. Heat the oil a small non-stick pan over a medium heat 2 minutes.

2. Add the De Costi Prawns to the pan and cook for 2 minutes then add the lemon & garlic butter for another 2 minutes.

3. Add the Prawns to the cooked pasta.

4. Toss through a handful of rocket. Garnish with fresh basil, sliced lemon and salt and pepper.

TIPS & HINTS:

Sprinkle with freshly grated parmesan for extra flavour.

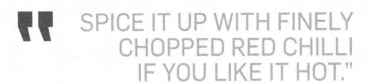 **❞ SPICE IT UP WITH FINELY CHOPPED RED CHILLI IF YOU LIKE IT HOT."**

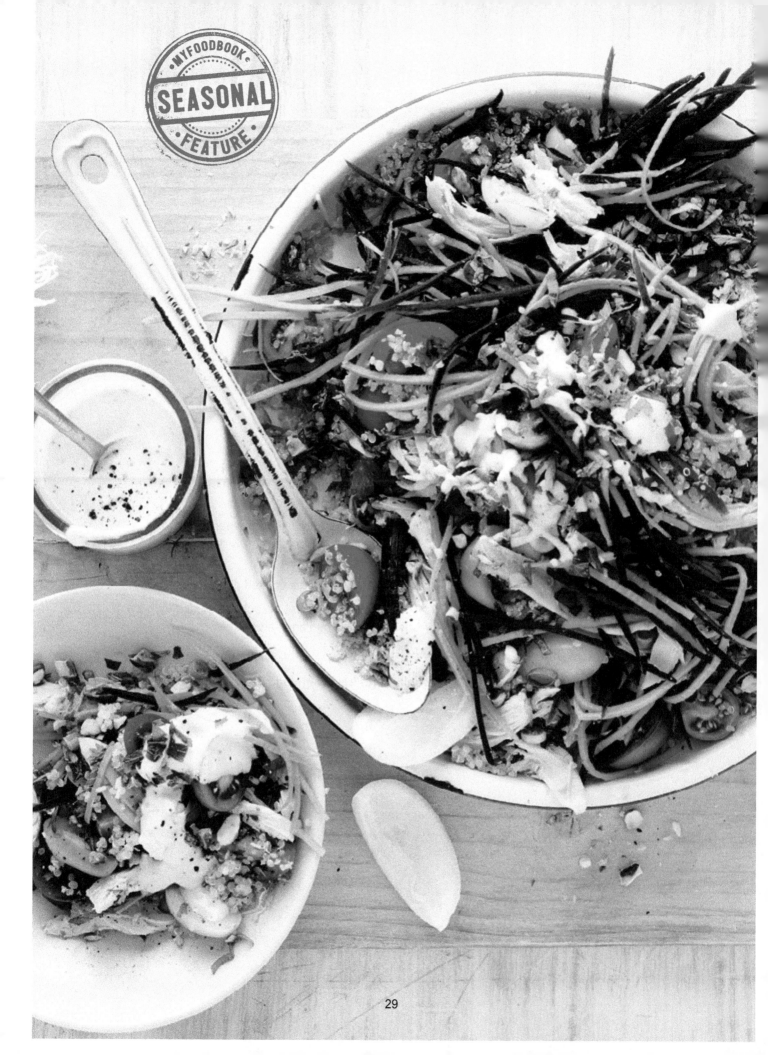

CARROT, TOMATO & CHICKEN QUINOA
salad

 PREP 20 MINS   **COOK** 30 MINS   **SERVES** 4-6

INGREDIENTS

1 cup white quinoa

1 small barbecued chicken

2 purple carrots

1 orange carrot

375g mixed baby tomatoes
(heirloom), quartered or halved

3 green onions (shallots), trimmed
and thinly sliced

½ cup small mint leaves, roughly
chopped

1 cup flat-leaf parsley leaves,
roughly chopped

½ cup shelled pistachio nuts,
roughly chopped

Lemon wedges, to serve

Lemon, tahini & yoghurt dressing

½ cup natural Greek-style yoghurt

1 tbs tahini

¼ cup lemon juice

METHOD

1. Place quinoa in a sieve and rinse in cold water.
    Combine quinoa and 2 cups water in medium
    saucepan and bring to the boil over medium-high
    heat. Reduce heat to low, cover and cook for
    15 minutes or until quinoa is cooked and water
    has been absorbed. Place quinoa into a large bowl.
    Set aside to cool slightly.

2. Meanwhile, shred chicken flesh, discarding skin and
    bones. Peel carrots. Using a julienne peeler or knife,
    shred carrots into long thin strips. Plunge carrots
    into a bowl of iced water. Stand for 5 minutes. Drain
    and pat dry carrots. Add chicken, carrots, tomatoes,
    green onions, mint, parsley and pistachios to quinoa.
    Toss to combine.

3. To make dressing, combine all ingredients in a bowl.
    Season with salt and pepper to taste. Whisk until
    well combined. Drizzle dressing over salad, gently
    toss and serve with lemon wedges.

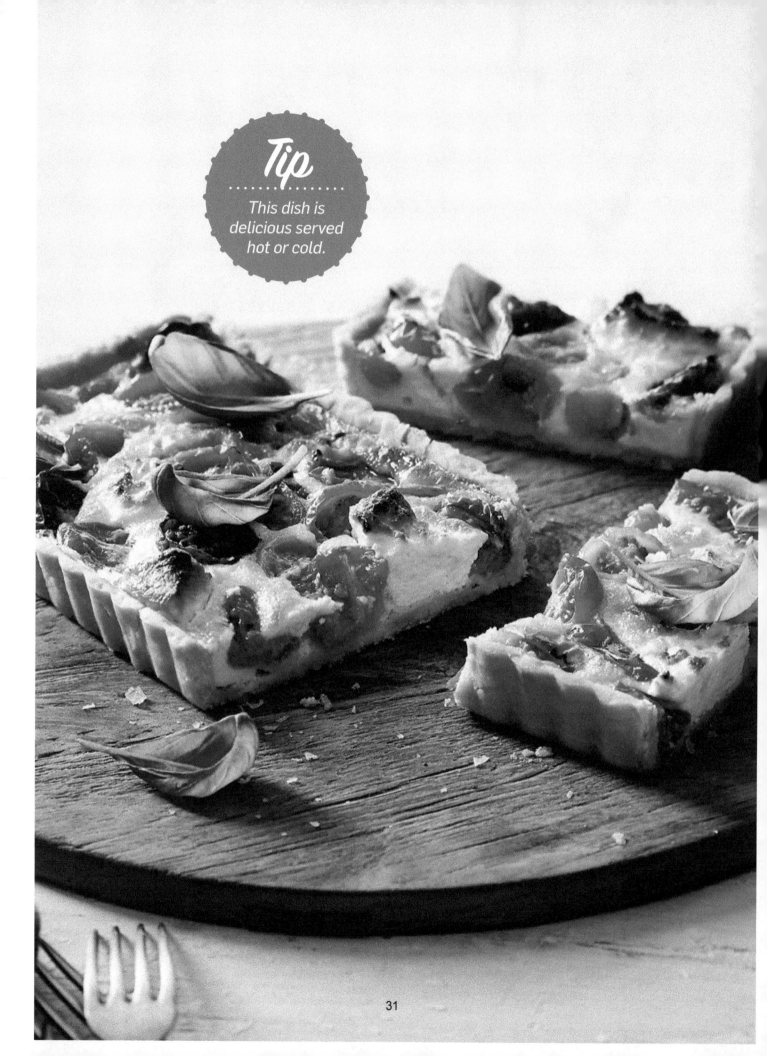

Tip

This dish is delicious served hot or cold.

TOMATO AND GOAT'S CHEESE
tart

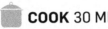 **PREP** 1 HOUR 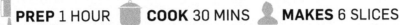 **COOK** 30 MINS **MAKES** 6 SLICES

INGREDIENTS

PASTRY

185g (1¼ cups) plain flour

¼ teaspoon baking powder

85g chilled Fairy margarine, cut into small pieces

1 egg yolk

1 tablespoon lemon juice

2–3 tablespoons cold water

FILLING

2 eggs

250 ml (1 cup) cream

Salt and pepper, to season

ASSEMBLY

250g cherry tomatoes, cut in half

150g goat's cheese

Basil leaves to garnish

METHOD

PASTRY

1. Combine flour, baking powder and Fairy in a food processor. Process until mixture resembles fine breadcrumbs. Add egg yolk, lemon juice and sufficient water until pastry comes together.

2. Knead lightly and pat into a round flat shape. Wrap in baking paper and place in the refrigerator for 30 minutes to rest.

3. Preheat oven to 200°C.

4. Roll dough out on a floured board and line a greased rectangular fluted fan tin.

5. Line with baking paper and fill with baking beans or rice. Rest in refrigerator for another 20 minutes.

6. Blind bake pastry for 10 minutes. Remove the paper and beans or rice, reduce the temperature to 180°C and bake for another 10 minutes or until golden.

FILLING

1. Lightly beat eggs and cream together, season with salt and pepper.

ASSEMBLY

1. Spread the cut tomatoes over the base and place chunks of goat's cheese over top.

2. Pour over the egg mix and bake for 10 minutes, reduce heat to 180°C and cook for a further 20 minutes or until filling is puffed and golden.

3. Top with fresh basil leaves to serve.

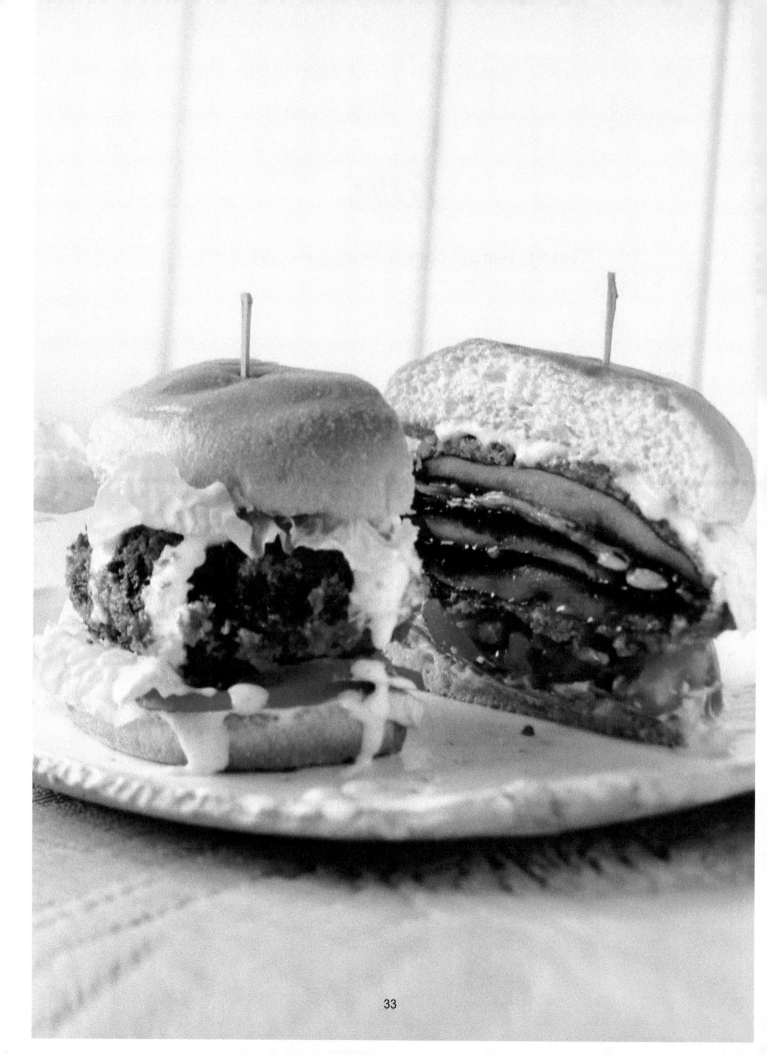

SOUTHERN-FRIED PORTABELLA MUSHROOM
burger

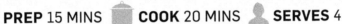

PREP 15 MINS   **COOK** 20 MINS   **SERVES** 4

INGREDIENTS

Vegetable oil or other neutral oil, for shallow frying, plus extra for cooking

12 Portabella Mushrooms, stems removed

100g mozzarella, sliced (optional)

75g (½ cup) plain flour

2 tsp mixed dried herbs

3 eggs, lightly beaten

1 ½ cups fresh breadcrumbs

Salt and pepper, to season

Brioche burger buns, lettuce, tomato and horseradish mustard mayonnaise, to serve

METHOD

1. In batches, heat 1 tbsp of oil over medium-low heat. Cook the mushrooms for 5 minutes each or until cooked through. Transfer to a plate and allow to cool

2. Place 4 mushrooms with the underside facing up, add a slice of mozzarella, if using, to each, then top each with a mushroom. Add another slice of mozzerella then top with the remaining mushrooms with the tops facing up

3. Place the flour, eggs and breadcrumbs into 3 separate bowls. Stir the mixed herbs through the flour and season well with salt and pepper. Dust the mushroom patties well in the flour, then dip in the eggs to coat, then repeat process and coat well in the breadcrumbs

4. Add enough oil into a deep frying pan to come 2cm up the sides and heat to 180°C. Shallow fry the mushroom burgers for 3 minutes each side or until golden. Remove and drain well on paper towel, then season with salt and pepper

5. Serve the mushroom steaks with salad or in a burger

TIPS & HINTS:

You can also use large flat white mushrooms, if you prefer

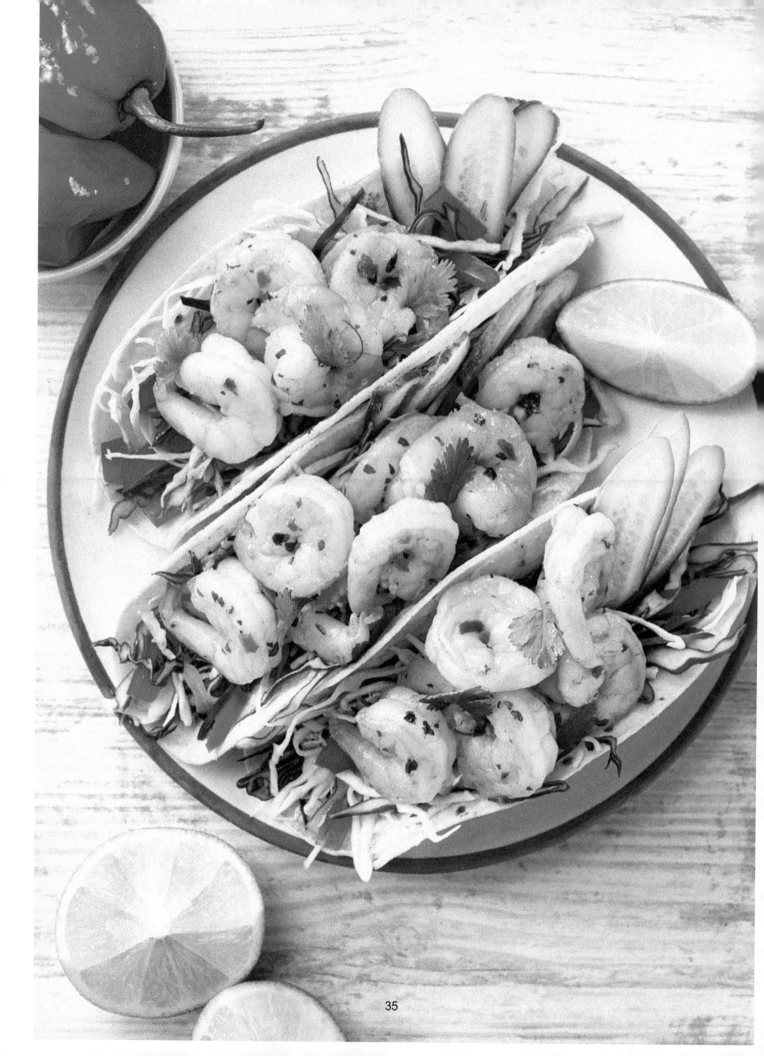

PRAWN SOFT
tortillas

 PREP 10 MINS **COOK** 8 MINS 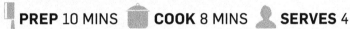 **SERVES** 4

INGREDIENTS

PRAWN TORTILLAS

1 x any of the De Costi Flavoured Prawn range

6 mini soft tortillas, warmed

2 cups red cabbage slaw, thinly chopped

1 small Lebanese cucumber, thinly sliced

TO SERVE

Lime wedges

METHOD

PRAWN TORTILLAS

1. Heat a non-stick pan over medium heat for 2 minutes. Add the De Costi Flavoured Prawns to the pan and heat 1 minute.

2. Toss the prawns in the pan for 2–3 minutes until sizzling and prawns change colour and are opaque.

TO SERVE

1. Lay the warmed tortillas on a flat surface and place a small amount of red cabbage slaw onto each tortilla.

2. Top with a spoonful of cooked sweet chilli prawns, garnish with sliced cucumber and wedges of lime.

TIPS & HINTS:

This dish is delicious served warm or cold. Add avocado to the base of the tortillas and sour cream to serve.

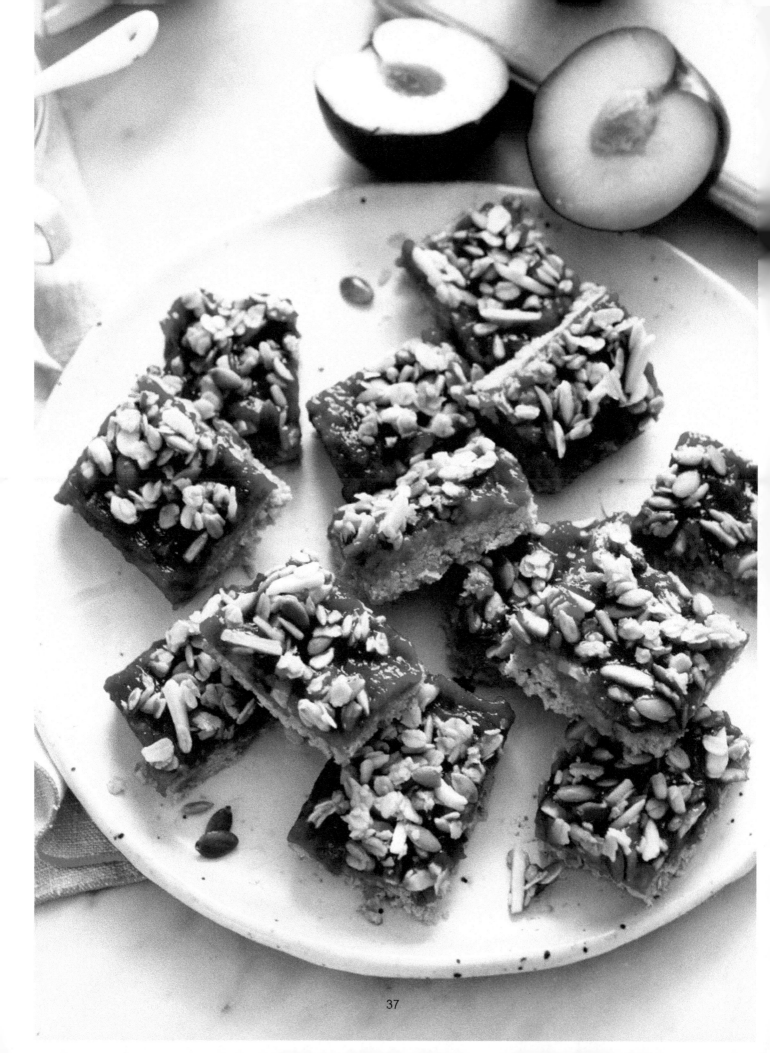

HEALTHY PLUM
slice

 PREP 20 MINS   **COOK** 55 MINS   👤 **MAKES** 12

INGREDIENTS

Filling

6 plums, stones removed, roughly chopped

2 tablespoons maple syrup

Base

2 cups rolled oats

1 cup almond meal

¼ cup maple syrup

2 tablespoons coconut oil

1 teaspoon sea salt flakes

1 teaspoon cinnamon

Topping

½ cup rolled oats

¼ cup slivered almonds

¼ cup pumpkin seeds

2 tablespoons sunflower seeds

1 tablespoon coconut oil

METHOD

Filling

1. Place plums and maple syrup into a saucepan and place over a medium heat. Bring mixture to the boil and simmer for 15-20 minutes until plums are soft, pulpy and firm. Cool. Place in fridge until required. (This can be made the day or night ahead of making.)

Base

1. Preheat oven to 180°C. Grease and line a 20cm x 20cm cake pan with baking paper.

2. To make the base place oats, almond meal, maple syrup, coconut oil, salt and cinnamon into a food processor and process until well combined and finely chopped. Press evenly over base of prepared cake pan. Bake for 15 minutes. Cool.

Topping

1. Spread plum mixture over cold base. For topping, combine oats, almonds, pumpkin seeds, sunflower seeds and coconut oil in a bowl. Stir until combined.

2. Sprinkle mixture over plums, pressing lightly. Bake for 20 minutes or until topping is light golden. Cool in pan. Remove from pan and cut into bars or squares.

3. Store in an airtight container in the refrigerator for up to 5 days.

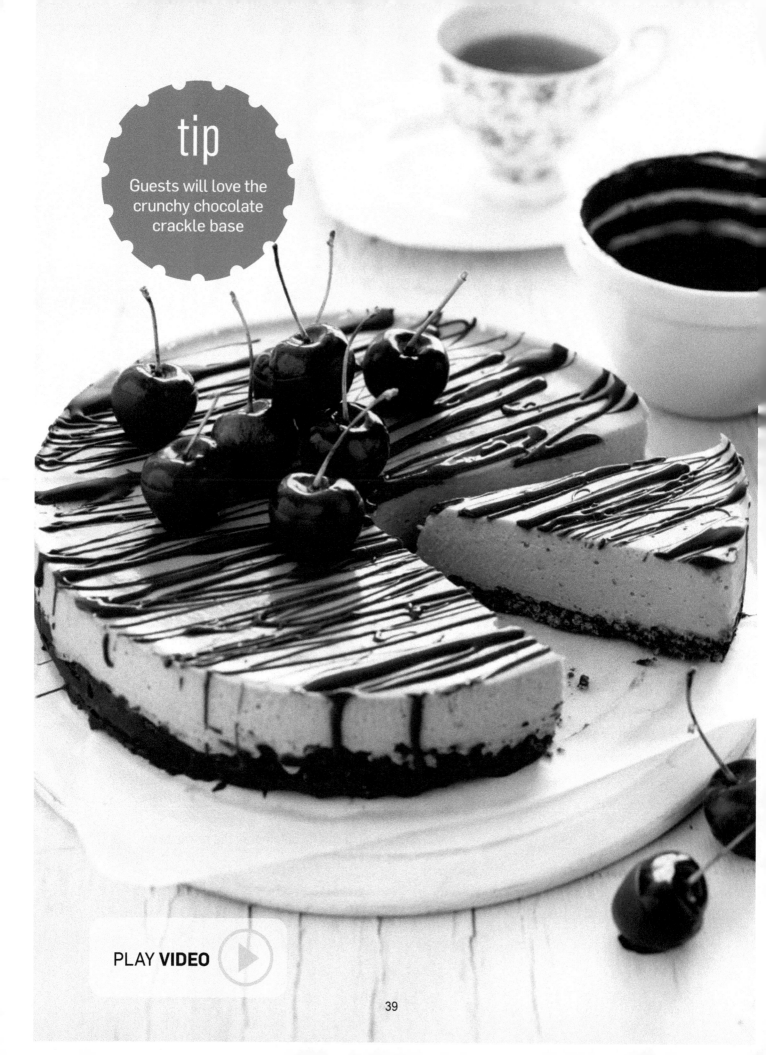

tip

Guests will love the crunchy chocolate crackle base

PLAY **VIDEO**

CHERRY COCONUT CHEESECAKE WITH
chocolate crackle base

PREP 30 MINS, PLUS 1 HOUR, 15 MINS SETTING TIME **SERVES** 12

INGREDIENTS

CHOCOLATE CRACKLE BASE

60g (¼ cup) Copha, chopped

60g dark chocolate, chopped

80g (½ cup) icing sugar mixture, sifted

2 tablespoons cocoa powder

50g (1 ⅔ cup) Kellogg's Rice Bubbles

20g (⅓ cup) desiccated coconut

CHEESECAKE FILLING

300g (1 ½ cups) cherries, pitted and halved

60ml (¼ cup) water

160g (1 cup) icing sugar mixture, sifted

500g cream cheese, chopped and softened

270ml can coconut cream

3 teaspoons powdered gelatine

CHOC-CHERRY TOPPING

100g dark chocolate, chopped

20g (1 tablespoon) Copha

12 cherries, extra

METHOD

CHOCOLATE CRACKLE BASE

1. Grease and line the base and sides of a 22cm spring form cake tin. In a heatproof bowl, combine chocolate and Copha. Place over a pot of lightly simmering water. Stir until melted. Remove from heat.

2. Place sugar, cocoa, rice bubbles and coconut in a large bowl. Add Copha mixture and mix to combine. Press into base of tin. Put in fridge to set for 10 minutes.

CHEESECAKE FILLING

3. Place cherries, sugar, water in a small saucepan over high heat. Bring to the boil and cook for 4 minutes, to soften. Remove from the heat and cool slightly for 5 minutes. Using a stick blender, blend until smooth.

4. Sprinkle over the gelatine and set aside for 5 minutes to dissolve. Mix until smooth. Set aside.

5. Place cheese in large bowl and using hand-held beaters, beat for 4 minutes until light and fluffy. Add coconut cream and beat for 4 minutes until light and smooth. Strain the cherry mixture through a sieve and gradually add to the cheese mixture. Stir to combine. Pour over base and put in fridge to set for 1 hour.

CHOC-CHERRY TOPPING

6. In a heatproof bowl, combine the chocolate and Copha. Place over a pot of lightly simmering water. Stir occasionally until melted. Remove from heat.

7. Half dip the cherries in the chocolate, place on baking paper and refrigerate for 2 minutes to set.

1. Remove cheesecake from tin and drizzle with chocolate mixture. Top with cherries to serve.

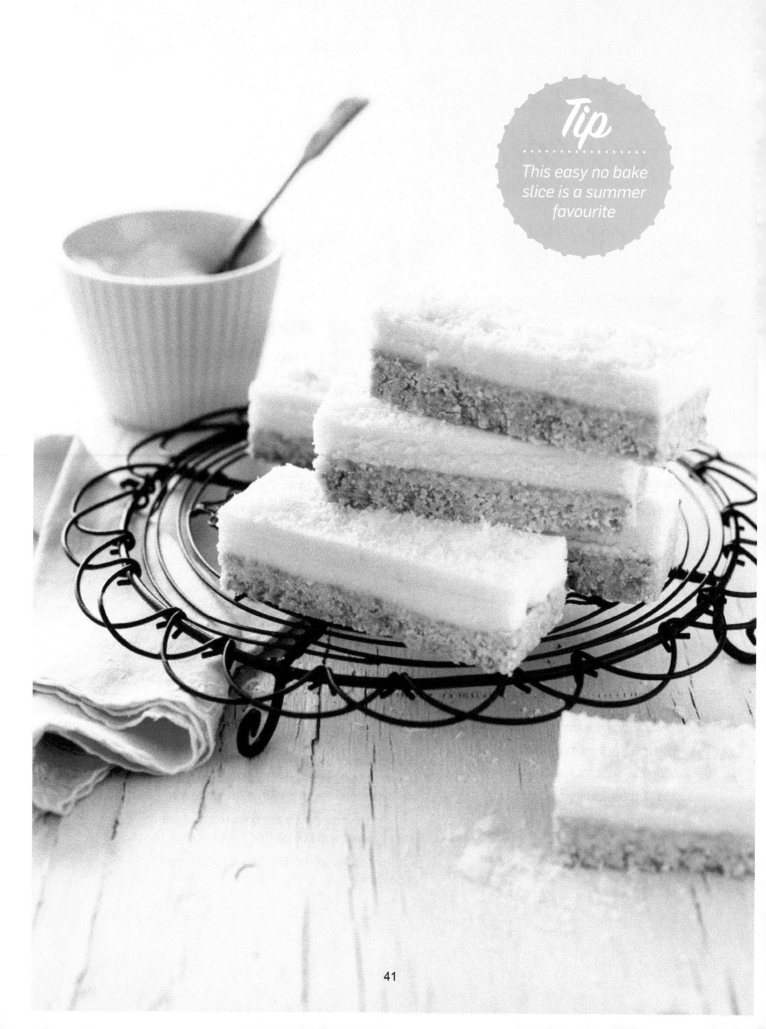

Tip

This easy no bake
slice is a summer
favourite

LEMON COCONUT
slice

 PREP 30 MINS   👤 **MAKES** 24 BARS

INGREDIENTS

BASE

125g (½ block) Copha, chopped

250g (1 packet) Arnott's Milk Coffee Biscuits

80g (1 cup) desiccated coconut

160g (½ cup) sweetened condensed milk

LEMON TOPPING

185g (¾ cup) Copha, chopped

110g (¾ cup) white chocolate melts

200g (⅔ cup) sweetened condensed milk

250g tub sour cream

60ml (¼ cup) lemon juice

2 teaspoons finely grated lemon rind

40g (½ cup) desiccated coconut, extra

1 teaspoon finely grated lemon rind, extra

METHOD

BASE

1. Grease and line a 20cm x 30cm slice tin. Make sure the paper has a 2cm overhang

2. Melt the Copha in a microwave on high or in a saucepan until fully melted. Using a food processor process the biscuits and coconut until they resemble fine breadcrumbs

3. Add the melted Copha and sweetened condensed milk and mix together. Press the biscuit mixture firmly into the tin, using the back of a spoon. Put in the fridge to set for 10 minutes

LEMON TOPPING

1. Melt the Copha and chocolate in a microwave on high or in a saucepan over low heat until fully melted and combined

2. Place sweetened condensed milk, sour cream, lemon juice and rind in a large bowl and mix to combine. Add the Copha chocolate mixture and mix until smooth

3. Pour over the base and smooth the top. Put in the fridge to set for 20 minutes

4. Place extra coconut and lemon rind in a small bowl and mix to combine. Sprinkle over the slice to serve. Slice into 24 bars

TIPS & HINTS

This slice will keep in an airtight container in the fridge for up to 3 days

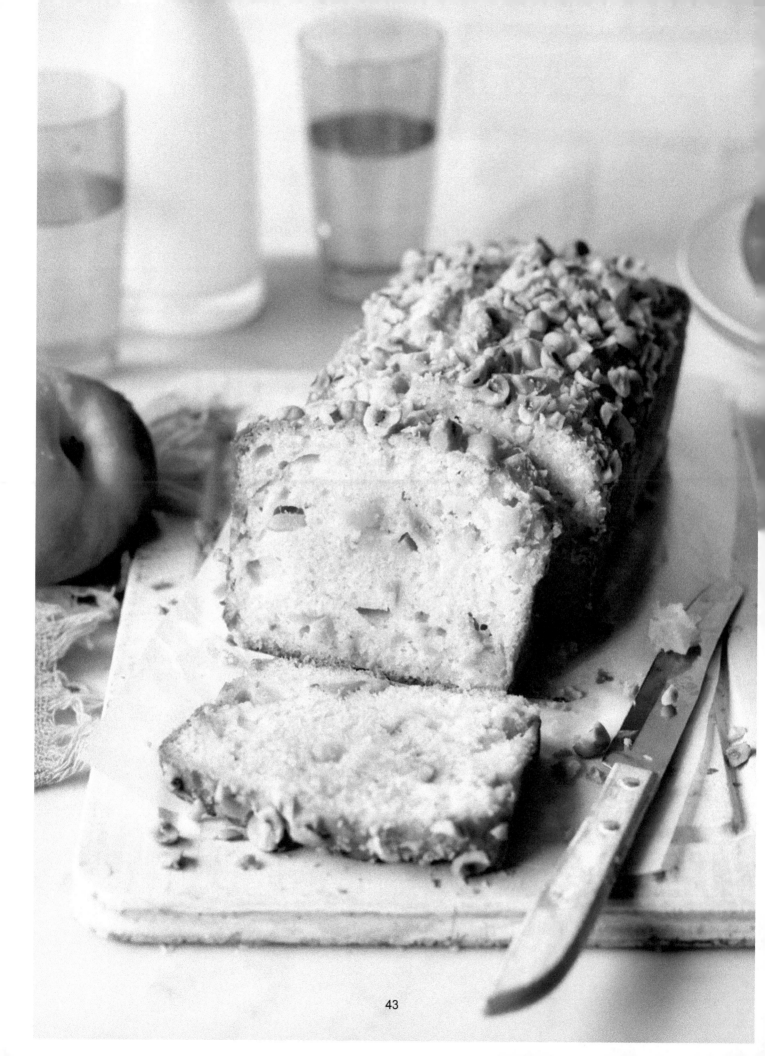

PEACH, COCONUT AND HAZELNUT *loaf*

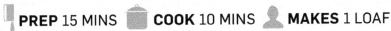 **PREP** 15 MINS **COOK** 10 MINS **MAKES** 1 LOAF

INGREDIENTS

125g butter, softened

⅔ cup caster sugar

1 teaspoon vanilla extract

2 eggs, at room temperature

1 cup sour cream

2 yellow peaches, stone removed, finely diced

1½ cups self-raising flour

½ cup plain flour

½ cup desiccated coconut

⅓ cup roasted hazelnuts, finely chopped

METHOD

1. Preheat oven to 180°C. Grease a 6 cup-capacity (20cm x 10cm x 7cm deep base measurement) loaf pan and line with baking paper, 5cm above line of pan. Using an electric mixer, beat butter, sugar and vanilla until pale and creamy. Add egg, 1 at a time, beating well after each addition.

2. Using a large metal spoon, gently fold in sour cream, peaches and coconut. Sift flours over batter and gently fold until combined.

3. Spoon batter into prepared loaf pan. Smooth top and sprinkle with chopped nuts, pressing gently into batter. Bake for 1 hour or until a skewer inserted into the centre comes out clean. Stand for 10 minutes before turning out onto a wire rack to cool.

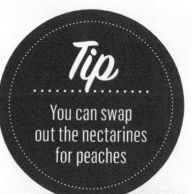

Tip

You can swap
out the nectarines
for peaches

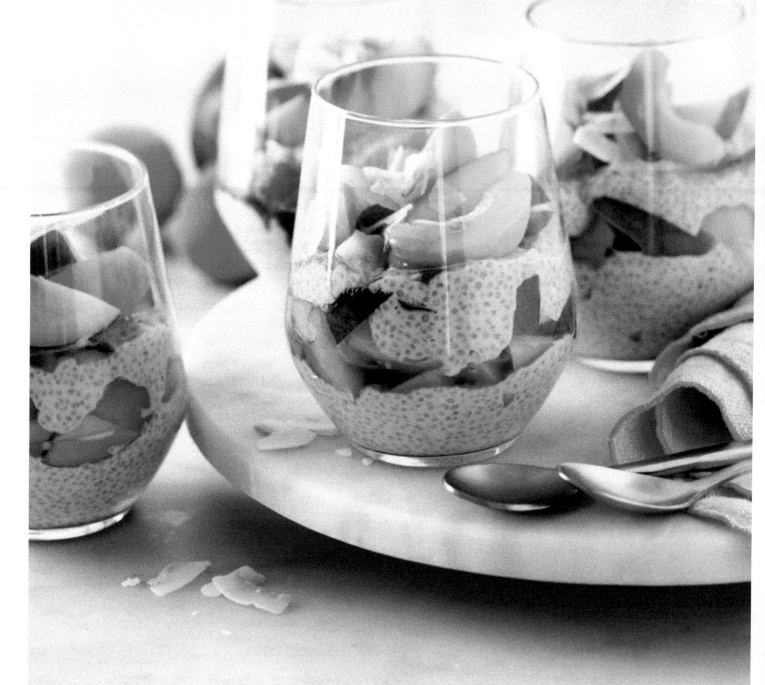

45

NECTARINE AND APRICOT COCONUT
chia puddings

PREP 25   **SERVES** 4

INGREDIENTS

2 x 270m cans coconut milk

¾ cup white chia seeds

1 teaspoon vanilla extract

4 yellow nectarines, stone removed, cut into thin wedges

4 apricots, stone removed, finely diced

½ cup maple syrup, to serve

¼ cup toasted flaked coconut, to serve

METHOD

1. Place coconut milk, chia seeds and vanilla into a bowl and stir until well combined. Set aside for 15 minutes to thicken.

2. Spoon half the chia mixture into the base of 4 x 1 cup-capacity glasses or glass bowls. Top with half the nectarines and apricots. Spoon remaining chia seed mixture over fruit. Place remaining fruit onto chia seed mixture.

3. Place in refrigerator for 1 hour or until cold. Drizzle the maple syrup over the fruit. Sprinkle with coconut and serve.

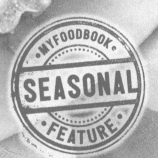

NO-BAKE BLUEBERRY & SWEET RICOTTA *tart*

PREP 25 MINS + CHILLING TIME **SERVES** 8

INGREDIENTS

Biscuit base

250g Butternut Snap or Marie biscuits

125g unsalted butter, melted

Ricotta cannoli filling

500g fresh ricotta

⅓ cup icing sugar, plus extra for dusting

½ tsp vanilla extract

250g blueberries

Finely shredded orange zest and honey, to serve

METHOD

1. To make the biscuit base, place biscuits into a food processor and process until finely chopped. Add butter and process until well combined.

2. Evenly press mixture into the base of 22cm wide x 2.5cm deep loose-base fluted tart pan. Refrigerate for 3 hours (or longer if time permits).

3. To make the filling, place ricotta, icing sugar and vanilla into a medium bowl. Using electric hand beaters, beat the mixture until smooth. Cover and chill until ready to serve.

4. Just before serving, fill the tart case with the ricotta mixture. Scatter with blueberries. Dust with icing sugar and sprinkle with orange zest. Drizzle with a little honey and serve.

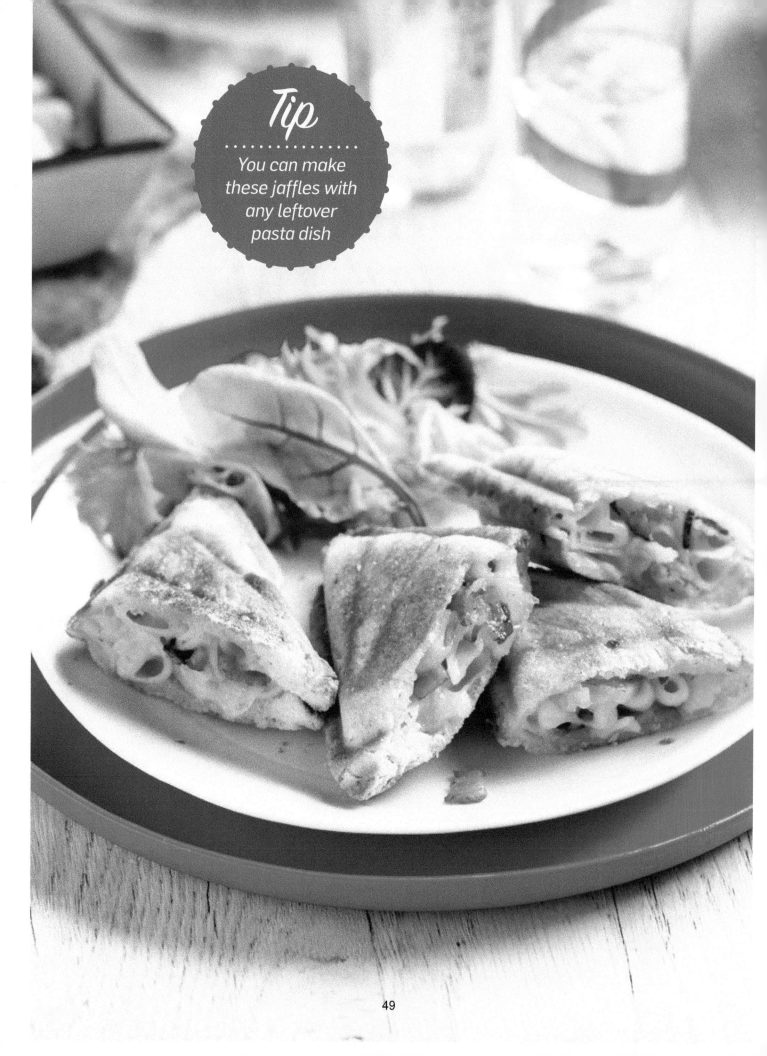

BACON MAC 'N' CHEESE
jaffles

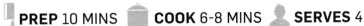 **PREP** 10 MINS   **COOK** 6-8 MINS   **SERVES** 4

INGREDIENTS

1 cup (320 g) leftover Bacon Mac 'N' Cheese

8 slices thick-cut white or wholemeal bread

4 tablespoons (80 g) Western Star Spreadable Original Soft

4 Bega Tasty Farmers' or Country Light Natural Cheese Slices

METHOD

1. Preheat a jaffle maker. Warm Mac 'N' Cheese slightly in your microwave

2. Spread bread on both sides with Western Star Spreadable Original Soft

3. Dividing mixture evenly, top 4 slices of bread with the Mac 'N' Cheese, spreading out leaving a 1 cm border. Top each sandwich with a Bega Tasty Farmers' Natural Cheese Slice and then top with the remaining bread

4. Cooking in 2 batches, place Mac 'N' Cheese filled bread into the jaffle maker and cook for 3-4 minutes until golden and toasted. Serve with a leafy green salad, if liked

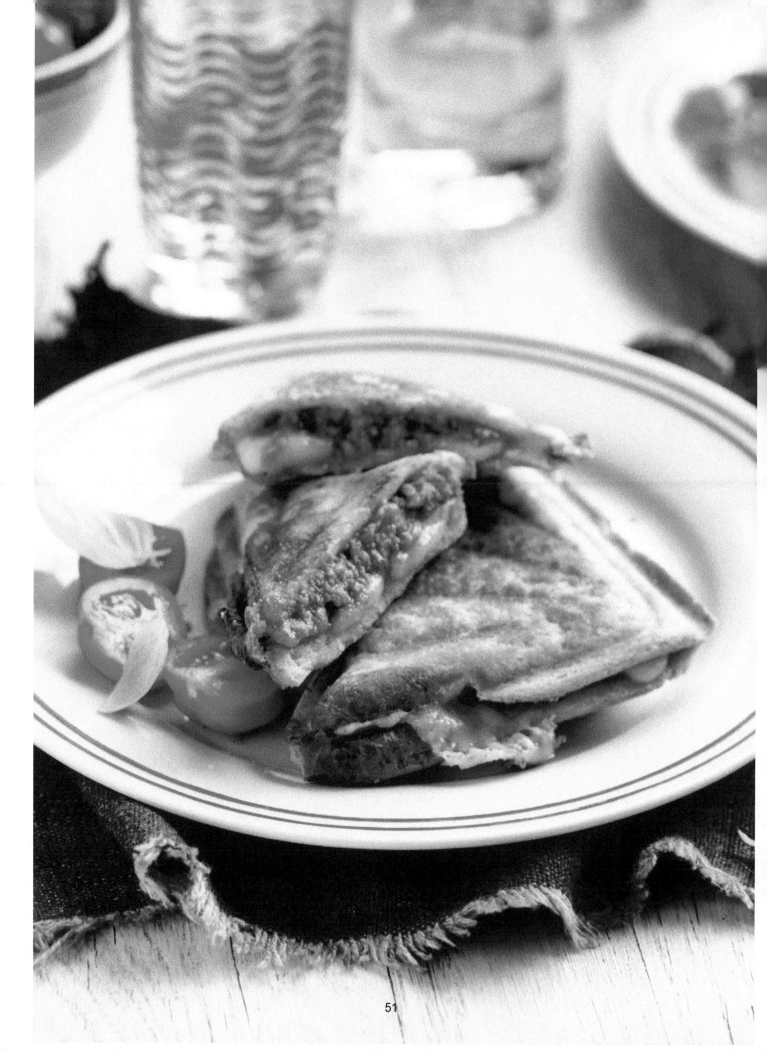

CHEESY BOLOGNESE *jaffles*

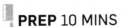 **PREP** 10 MINS 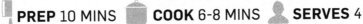 **COOK** 6-8 MINS   **SERVES** 4

INGREDIENTS

1⅓ cups (330 g) leftover Bolognese sauce

8 slices thick-cut white or wholemeal bread

4 tablespoons (80 g) Western Star Spreadable Original Soft

8 Bega Tasty Farmers' or Country Light Natural Cheese Slices

METHOD

1. Preheat a jaffle maker. Warm leftover Bolognese sauce slightly in your microwave

2. Spread each piece of bread on both sides with Western Star Spreadable Original Soft

3. Dividing mixture evenly, top 4 slices of bread with the Bolognese sauce, spreading out leaving a 1 cm border. Top each sandwich with 2 Bega Tasty Farmers' Natural Cheese Slices, and then top with the remaining bread

4. Cooking in 2 batches, place Bolognese-filled bread into the jaffle maker and cook for 3-4 minutes until golden and toasted. Serve with a side salad, if liked

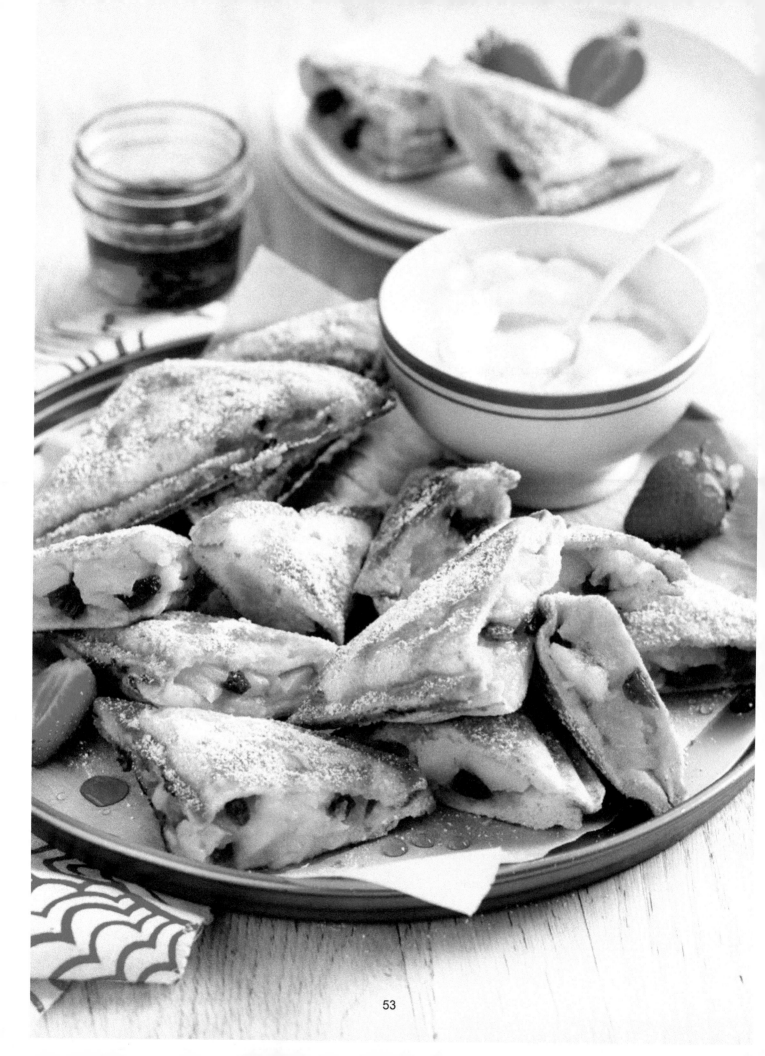

TRADITIONAL HOT APPLE PIE

jaffles

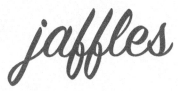

 PREP 12 MINS **COOK** 6-8 MINS   **SERVES** 4

INGREDIENTS

*300 mL Western Star
Thickened Cream*

2 cups canned pie fruit sliced apples

¼ cup sultanas

½ teaspoon ground cinnamon

Good pinch allspice

*8 slices thick-cut white or
wholemeal bread*

*4 tablespoons (80 g) Western Star
Spreadable Original Soft*

Icing sugar, for dusting

Maple syrup, for drizzling

METHOD

1. Using an electric hand mixer, whip Western Star Thickened Cream in a bowl until soft peaks form. Set aside

2. Preheat a jaffle maker. Combine apples, sultanas, cinnamon and allspice in a bowl

3. Spread bread on both sides with Western Star Spreadable Original Soft

4. Dividing mixture evenly, top 4 slices of bread with the apple mixture, spreading out leaving a 1 cm border. Top with the remaining bread

5. Cooking in 2 batches, place apple-filled bread into the jaffle maker and cook for 3-4 minutes until golden and toasted

6. Dust with icing sugar and serve with whipped cream and a drizzle of maple syrup. Scatter with fresh strawberries, if liked

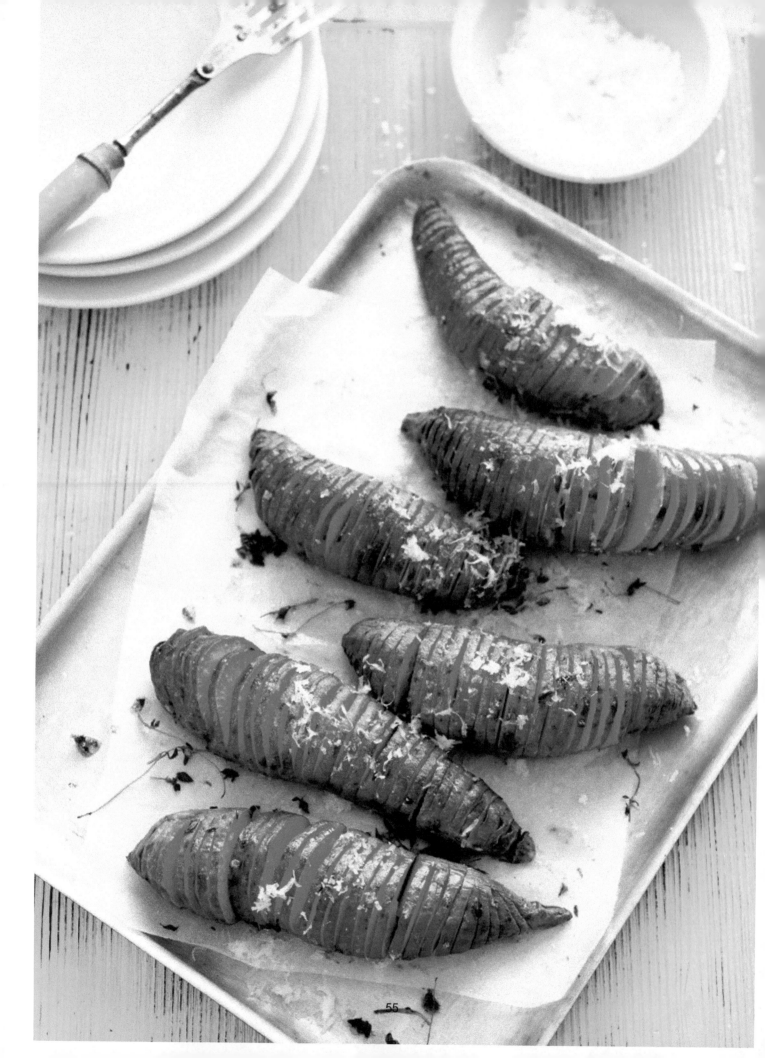

HASSELBACK
sweet potatoes

 PREP 15 MINS   **COOK** 1 HOUR 10 MINS   **MAKES** 6

INGREDIENTS

6 x 200g Sweet Potatoes, scrubbed

6 sprigs fresh thyme, plus extra for serving

Olive oil

¼ teaspoon sea salt

⅓ cup finely grated parmesan

METHOD

1. Preheat oven to 200°C/180°C. Carefully cut 3mm slices into the sweet potatoes, leaving 5mm intact at the bottom. Place on a baking-paper lined oven tray

2. Strip the leaves from the thyme and tuck in between the fans of the sweet potatoes

3. Drizzle with oil and sprinkle with salt

4. Bake for 1 hour -1 hour 10 minutes until golden and soft in the middle when easily pierced with a knife. Serve sprinkled with parmesan

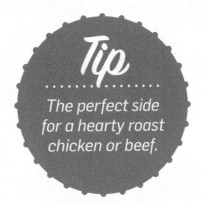

Tip

The perfect side for a hearty roast chicken or beef.

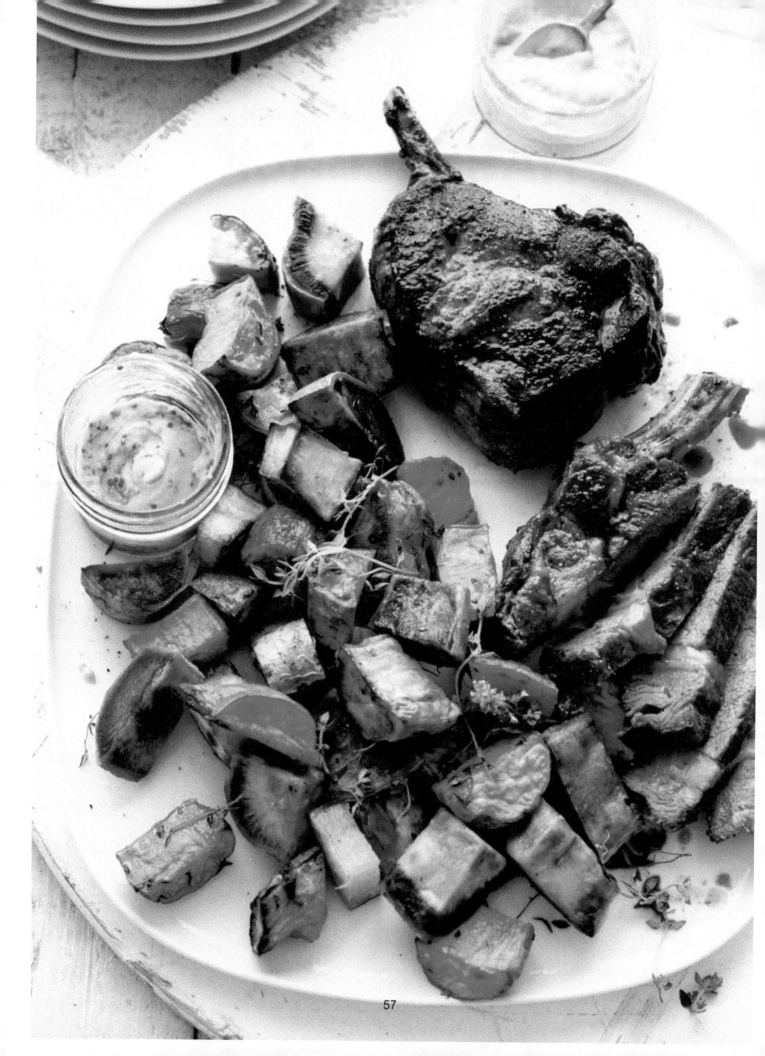

ROAST SWEET POTATO MEDLEY
with rib-eye steak

 PREP 10 MINS **COOK** 50 MINS 👤 **SERVES** 4

INGREDIENTS

400g each Gold, Purple and White Sweet Potato, chopped

3 tablespoons olive oil, plus extra for steaks

½ bunch fresh thyme sprigs

4 x beef rib-eye steaks

Mustard, to serve

METHOD

1. Preheat oven to 200°C/180°C. Line two oven trays with baking paper. Combine sweet potatoes evenly on trays. Toss with olive oil to coat and season. Bake for 35-40 minutes until golden and tender

2. Meanwhile, drizzle steaks with extra oil. Sprinkle both sides with salt and pepper. Cook steaks in a large oven-proof frying pan over medium-high heat for 2-3 minutes each side until browned. Transfer pan to oven and cook for about 5 minutes until cooked to taste. Rest steaks for 5 minutes

3. Serve steaks with potato medley and mustard

TIP: *Twist it by serving the rib-eye steaks with hasselback sweet potatoes for dinner party wow or with sweet potato mash for when time is of the essence.*

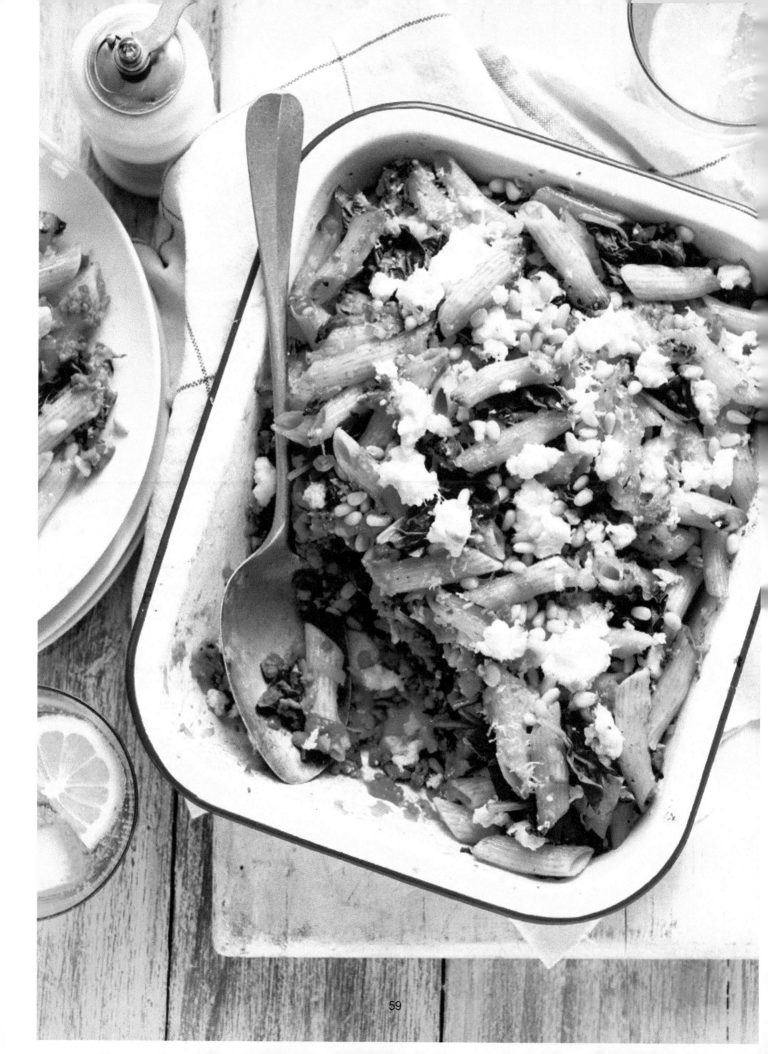

SWEET POTATO PASTA BAKE WITH
spinach and pine nuts

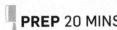 **PREP** 20 MINS 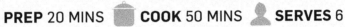 **COOK** 50 MINS   **SERVES** 6

INGREDIENTS

350g penne or other pasta

1 tablespoon olive oil

1 small onion, finely chopped

2 garlic cloves, crushed

500g lean beef mince

400g Sweet Potato, peeled, coarsely grated

1 small zucchini, coarsely grated

2 tablespoons tomato paste

400g can diced tomatoes

1 cup salt-reduced beef stock

4 sprigs thyme

50g baby spinach leaves

100g ricotta

½ cup (40g) grated parmesan

2 tablespoons pine nuts

METHOD

1. Cook pasta in a large pan of salted, boiling water until al dente. Drain well

2. Meanwhile, heat oil in a medium pan on medium-high heat. Cook onion and garlic for 3-4 minutes until softened. Add beef and cook until browned, breaking up lumps with a spoon. Add sweet potato and zucchini. Cook for 2 minutes until softened slightly

3. Add paste, tomatoes, stock and thyme. Simmer, uncovered for 15-20 minutes until thickened slightly. Stir through spinach leaves until wilted

4. Meanwhile, preheat oven to 220°C/200°C fan-forced

5. Combine pasta and beef mixture in an 8-cup capacity ovenproof dish. Sprinkle with ricotta, parmesan and pine nuts. Bake for 15-20 minutes until golden

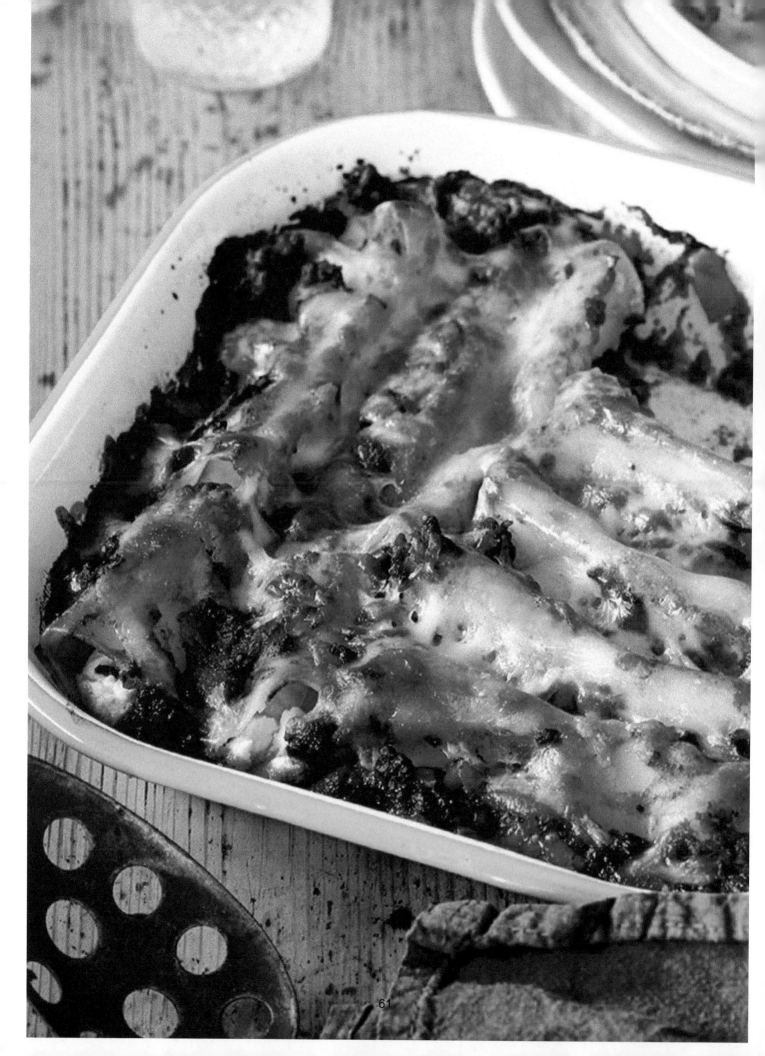

RICOTTA CANNELLONI
bolognese bake

 PREP 10 MINS 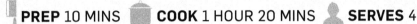 **COOK** 1 HOUR 20 MINS   **SERVES** 4

INGREDIENTS

2 tbsp olive oil

500g quality minced beef

1 brown onion, finely chopped

2 garlic cloves, finely chopped

1 carrot, peeled and finely chopped

2 celery sticks, finely chopped

2 x tins whole peeled tomatoes

200ml red wine (or water)

1 x 500g tub Perfect Italiano Ricotta

Zest of 1 lemon

200g cannelloni

150g Perfect Italiano Grated Perfect Bakes Cheese

METHOD

1. Heat the oil in a large pan over a medium heat. Once hot, add the mince and use a wooden spoon to break up. Continue to stir and cook for 5 minutes or until the mince has browned. Add the onion, garlic, carrot and celery and continue to cook for 10 minutes or until the vegetables have softened. Add the tomatoes and wine (or water) and stir, breaking up tomatoes with the back of the wooden spoon. Bring the mixture to a simmer and then reduce the heat to low. Simmer for 30 minutes, stirring regularly. Season to taste and set aside to cool slightly

2. Preheat the oven to 180°C

3. To prepare the cannelloni, mix the Perfect Italiano Ricotta with the lemon zest, and then season with salt and pepper. Carefully fill the cannelloni with the ricotta using a knife or piping bag

4. Spoon half of the Bolognese into a large baking dish and then gently lay the filled cannelloni into the dish. Top the cannelloni with the remaining Bolognese and then sprinkle over the Perfect Italiano Perfect Bakes Cheese. Place the dish into the oven and bake for 35 minutes or until golden and bubbling

5. Remove from the oven, and allow to sit for 5 minutes before serving

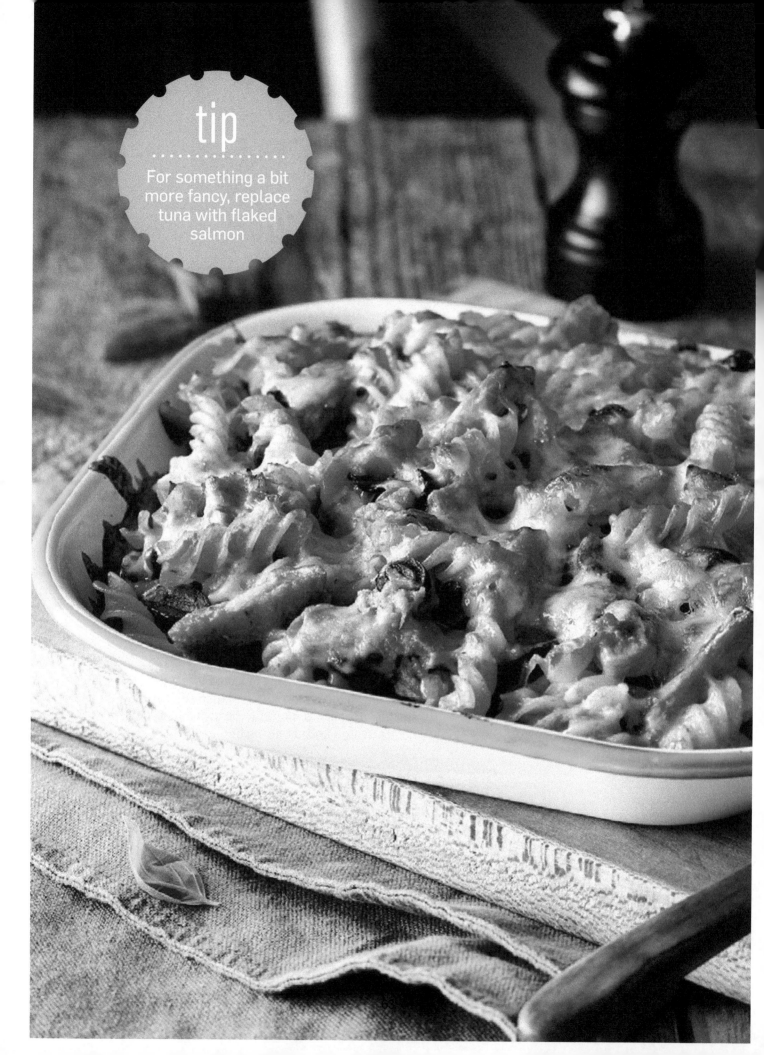

tip

....

For something a bit
more fancy, replace
tuna with flaked
salmon

TUNA, TOMATO AND MOZZARELLA
fusilli bake

 PREP 5 MINS   **COOK** 35 MINS   **SERVES** 4

INGREDIENTS

400g fusilli

1 tbsp olive oil

2 garlic cloves, sliced

400g tomato passata

425g chopped tomatoes

10 basil leaves, torn

⅓ cup pitted kalamata olives, chopped

1 x 425g tin tuna in spring water, drained and flaked

200g Perfect Italiano Mozzarella Cheese

METHOD

1. Cook the fusilli according to packet instructions, drain and set aside

2. Preheat the oven to 180°C

3. Heat the olive oil in a large deep-sided pan over a medium heat. Add the garlic and fry for 1 minute before adding the passata and chopped tomatoes. Bring to a simmer and then reduce the heat to low. Add the basil and olives and mix well. Continue to simmer for 5 minutes and then season with salt and pepper to taste

4. Add the drained pasta and tuna to the sauce, and mix well to coat the pasta and break up tuna. Transfer the mixture to a baking dish and sprinkle over the Perfect Italiano Mozzarella. Carefully place in the oven to bake for 20-25 minutes or until golden brown

5. Remove from the oven and allow to sit for 5 minutes before serving

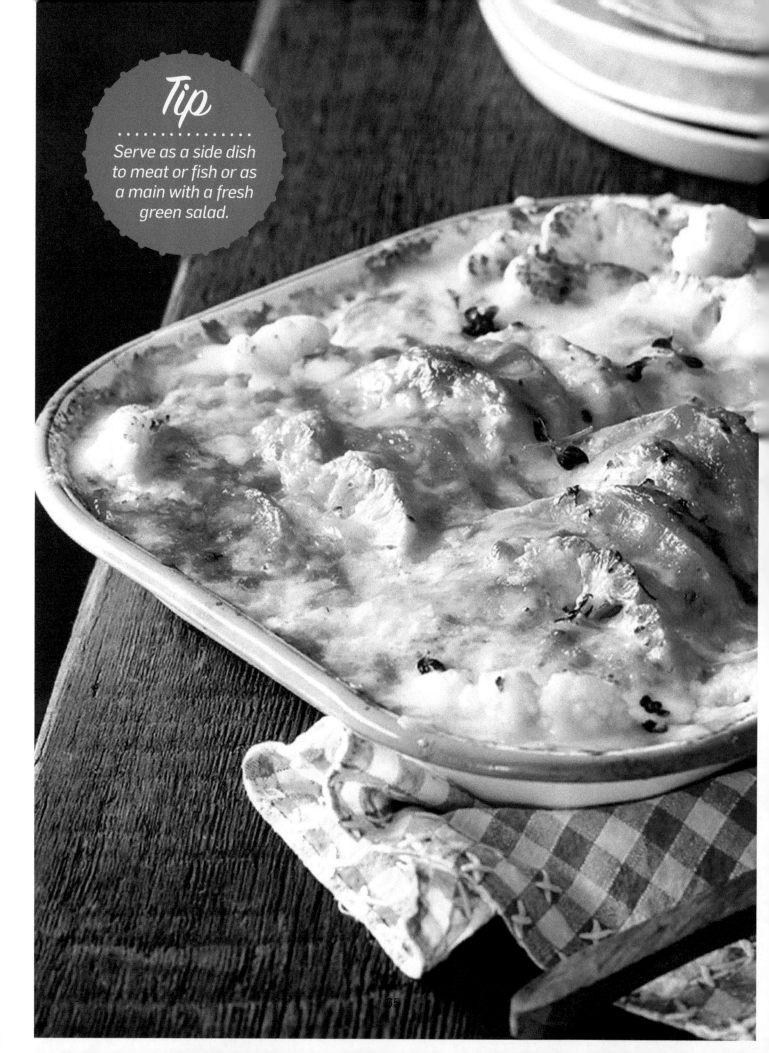

Tip

Serve as a side dish
to meat or fish or as
a main with a fresh
green salad.

CREAMY
SWEET POTATO
cauliflower bake

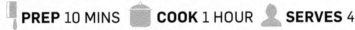 **PREP** 10 MINS **COOK** 1 HOUR **SERVES** 4

INGREDIENTS

400g sweet potato, peeled and sliced into 1cm slices

¼ head cauliflower, cut into 2cm slices

200ml cream

200ml milk

2 garlic cloves, peeled

⅓ cup Perfect Italiano Grated Parmesan

4 sprigs thyme, leaves removed

250g Perfect Italiano Perfect Bakes

METHOD

1. Preheat the oven to 180°C

2. Arrange the sweet potato and cauliflower into the dish so that the vegetables fit snuggly

3. Combine the cream, milk and garlic in a small saucepan and place over a low heat. Bring to a simmer and then turn off the heat. Stir through the Perfect Italiano Parmesan and the thyme, and then season with salt and pepper. Set aside for a couple of minutes before removing the garlic cloves

4. Carefully pour the cream mixture over the vegetables and then cover the baking dish with foil. Place into the oven to bake for 30 minutes

5. Remove from the oven and sprinkle over the Perfect Italiano Perfect Bakes. Return to the oven uncovered for a further 30 minutes or until golden. The vegetables should be tender when pierced with a knife

6. Remove from the oven and serve

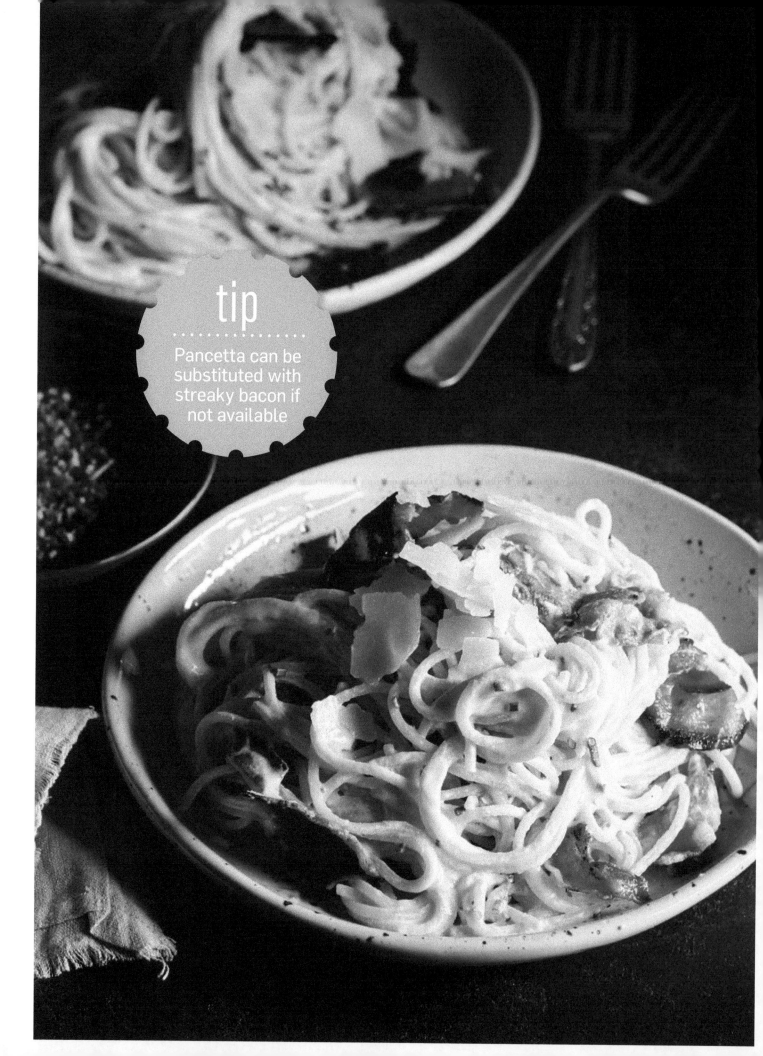

tip

Pancetta can be substituted with streaky bacon if not available

SPAGHETTI WITH CRISPY PANCETTA
with four cheese ricotta

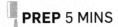 **PREP** 5 MINS **COOK** 10 MINS 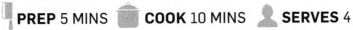 **SERVES** 4

INGREDIENTS

500g spaghetti

1 tbsp olive oil

4 slices pancetta, chopped

450g   Ricotta Pasta
Stir Through, Four Cheese

Salt and Pepper to taste

⅓ cup chives, finely chopped,
to garnish

Perfect Italiano Shaved Parmesan,
to serve

METHOD

1. Cook pasta according to packet instructions

2. Meanwhile, add olive oil to a large pan and place over medium to high heat. Once hot add the pancetta and fry until crispy and golden. Turn heat to low and add drained cooked pasta to the pan

3. Add   Ricotta Pasta Stir Through, Four Cheese to the pot and gently stir through

4. Once warmed through, season to taste and garnish with chives and Perfect Italiano Shaved Parmesan

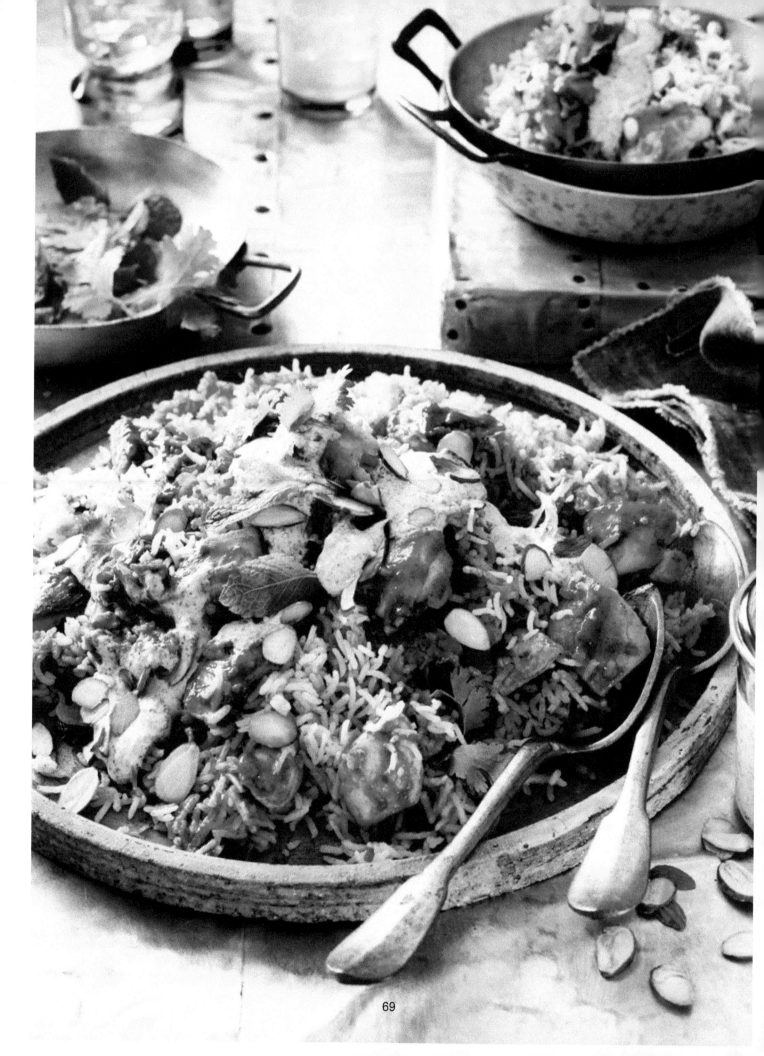

CHICKEN BIRYANI WITH CREAMY CORIANDER
and mint sauce

 PREP 10 MINS   **COOK** 55 MINS **SERVES** 4

INGREDIENTS

1 cup thick plain yoghurt

½ cup mint leaves, roughly chopped

½ cup coriander leaves, roughly chopped

1 lemon, juiced

2 cups basmati rice

1 tablespoon vegetable oil

1 brown onion, diced

500g chicken thigh fillets, diced

375g Passage to India Biryani simmer sauce

⅓ cup sultanas

Toasted natural flaked almonds, to serve

Coriander sprigs, to serve

METHOD

1. Place yoghurt, mint leaves and coriander leaves into a small food processor and pulse until a smooth pale green sauce forms. Transfer to a bowl. Stir through ¼ cup lemon juice, salt and white pepper

2. Rinse rice until water runs clear. Place into a medium saucepan and cover with water. Place over a high heat and bring to the boil. Reduce heat to low, cover and cook for 8 minutes. Drain

3. Heat oil in a frying pan over a medium high heat. Add onion and chicken and cook for 8 minutes or until browned. Pour Passage to India Biryani simmer sauce over chicken and bring to the boil. Reduce heat to low and simmer for 10 minutes

4. Sprinkle sultanas over chicken mixture. Spoon rice evenly over chicken and sultanas. Cover with a sheet of baking paper, tucking into side of pan. Cover and cook for 10 minutes. Remove from heat and stand for 10 minutes. Sprinkle with toasted almonds. Serve with coriander & mint sauce and coriander sprigs

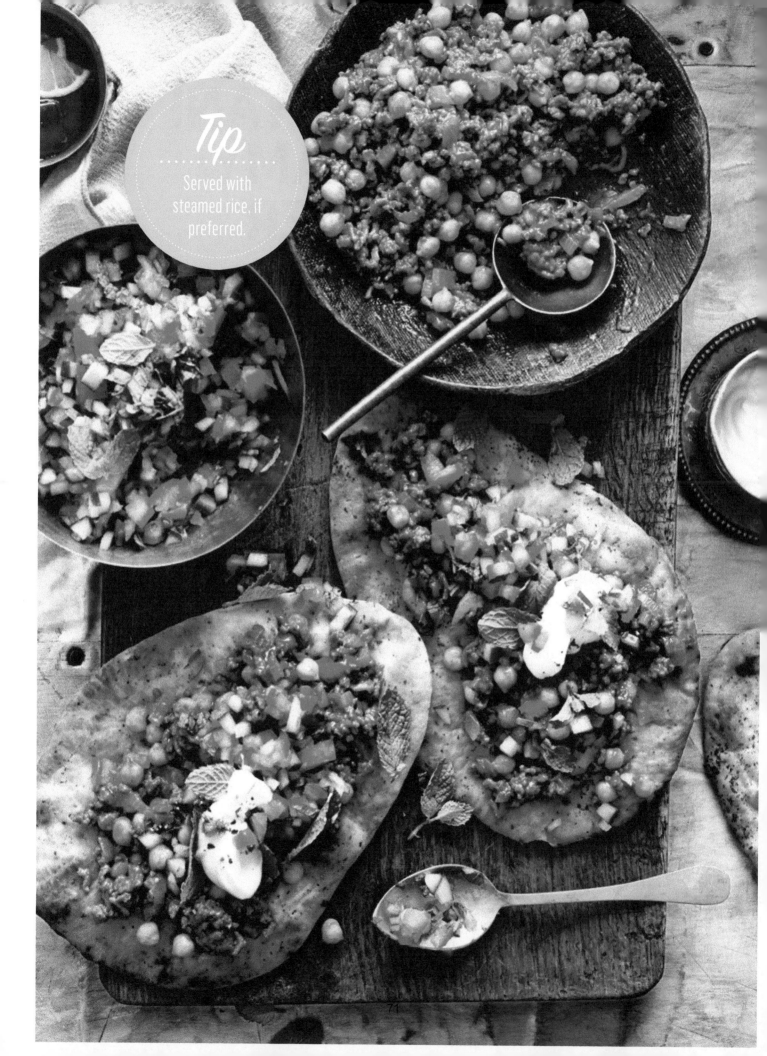

Tip

Served with
steamed rice, if
preferred.

MINCE AND
chickpea curry

 PREP 15 MINS **COOK** 25 MINS 👤 **SERVES** 4

INGREDIENTS

1 tablespoon vegetable oil

1 brown onion, diced

500g beef mince

375g Passage to India Mild Mince
Curry simmer sauce

400g can chickpeas, drained, rinsed

3 tomatoes, seeds removed,
finely diced

1 Lebanese cucumber, seeds
removed, finely diced

1 small red onion, finely diced

1 lemon, finely grated rind and
¼ cup juice

¼ cup finely chopped mint

Naan or Roti bread, warmed, to
serve

Thick plain yoghurt, to serve

Mint sprigs, to serve

METHOD

1. Heat oil in a deep frying pan over medium heat. Add
   onion and cook for 5 minutes or until softened. Add
   mince and stir with a wooden spoon to break up
   mince. Cook for 8 minutes or until browned. Pour
   Passage to India Mild Mince Curry simmer sauce
   over mince and stir until well combined. Bring to the
   boil, reduce heat to low and cook for 15 minutes or
   until slightly thickened. Stir through chickpeas. Cook
   for 2 minutes or until heated through. Season with
   salt and pepper

2. Meanwhile, combine tomato, cucumber, red onion,
   lemon rind, lemon juice and mint in a bowl. Prepare
   bread as per packet instructions

3. Place a naan or roti bread onto each serving plate.
   Top with curried mince, tomato & mint sambal, a
   dollop of yoghurt and mint sprigs. Serve immediately

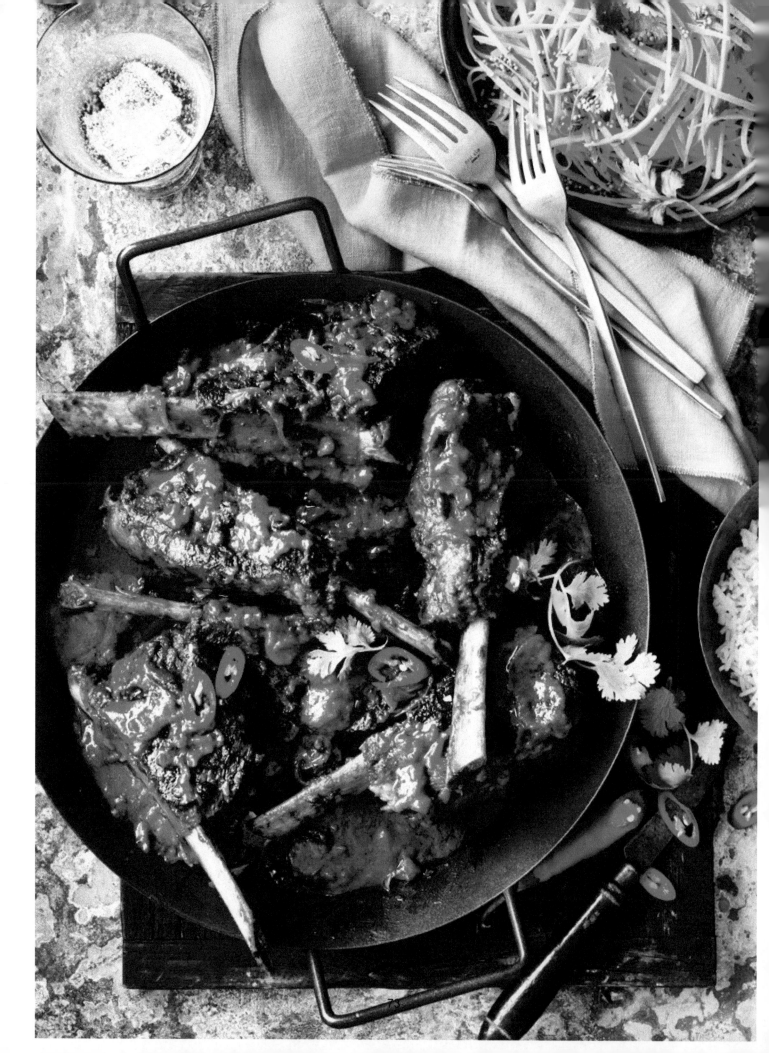

SPICY VINDALOO
beef ribs

 PREP 10 MINS   **COOK** 1.5 HOURS **SERVES** 4

INGREDIENTS

1.2kg beef ribs

2 tablespoons vegetable oil

2 small red onion, cut into thin wedges

375g Passage to India Vindaloo simmer sauce

2 teaspoons mustard seeds

1 teaspoon cumin seeds

3 carrots, shredded

⅓ cup coriander leaves, plus extra to serve

Steamed basmati rice, to serve

Finely sliced red chilli, to serve (optional)

METHOD

1. Place ribs into a saucepan and cover with cold water. Place over a high heat and bring to the boil. Reduce heat and simmer for 25 minutes. Remove from heat and cool in liquid. Drain. Cut ribs into smaller pieces

2. Heat half the oil in a deep frying pan over medium heat. Add half the onion and cook for 3 minutes or until softened. Add Passage to India Vindaloo simmer sauce and bring to the boil. Add beef ribs and stir until coated with sauce. Reduce heat to low, cover and simmer for 1 hour or until beef is tender

3. Meanwhile, heat remaining oil in a frying pan over medium heat. Add remaining onion and cook for 3 minutes or until softened. Add mustard seeds and cumin seeds. Cook for 2 minutes or until aromatic. Add carrots and cook for 3 minutes or until just softened. Remove from heat and season with salt and white pepper. Stir through coriander leaves just before serving. Spoon rice onto serving plates. Top with ribs and sauce and serve with carrot salad, extra coriander and chilli, if you like

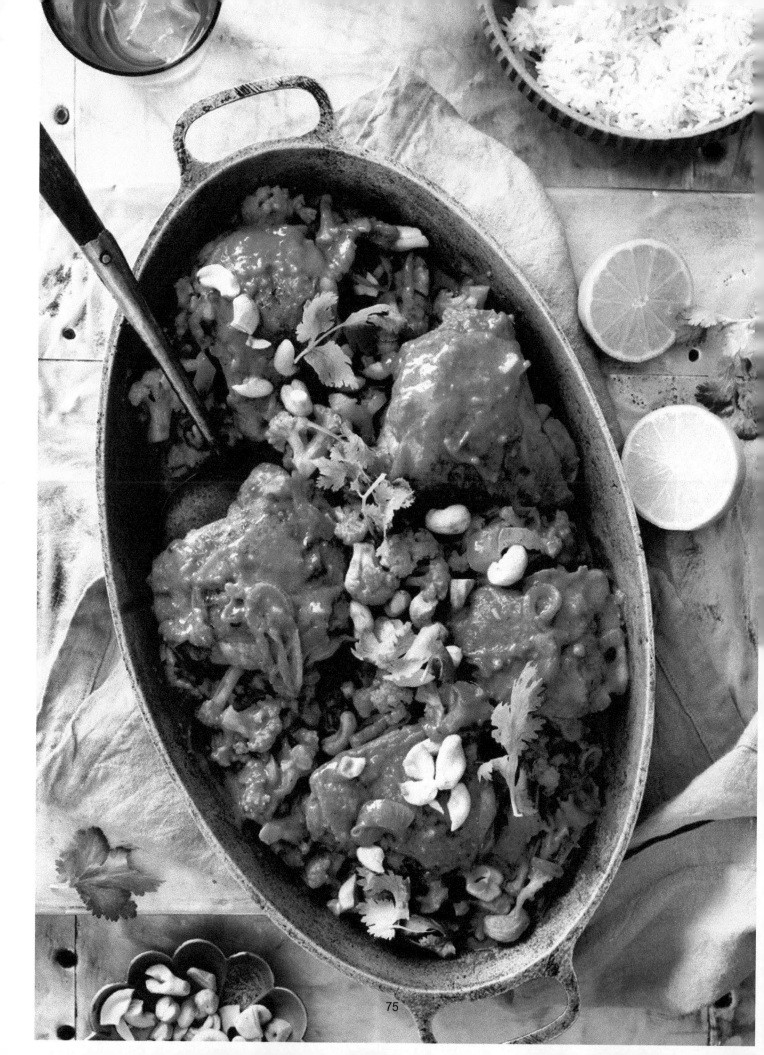

ONE-PAN BUTTER CHICKEN
with cauliflower

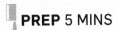 **PREP** 5 MINS 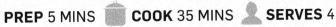 **COOK** 35 MINS **SERVES** 4

INGREDIENTS

1 tablespoon vegetable oil

8 chicken thigh cutlets, with skin on

1 brown onion, thinly sliced

½ (500g) cauliflower, cut into florets

375g Passage to India Butter Chicken Simmer Sauce

Steamed basmati rice, to serve

Roasted salted cashews, roughly chopped, to serve

Coriander sprigs, to serve

METHOD

1. Heat oil in a large non-stick frying pan over medium heat. Add chicken pieces and cook for 10 minutes or until browned on all sides. Transfer to a plate. Drain excess fat and discard

2. Add onion and cauliflower to pan and cook for 5 minutes or until softened. Pour Passage to India Butter Chicken Simmer Sauce over vegetables and bring to a simmer. Return chicken pieces to pan, coating well with sauce. Cover pan, reduce heat and simmer for 20 minutes or until chicken is cooked through.

3. Spoon rice onto a platter. Top with chicken, vegetables and sauce. Sprinkle with cashew nuts and coriander

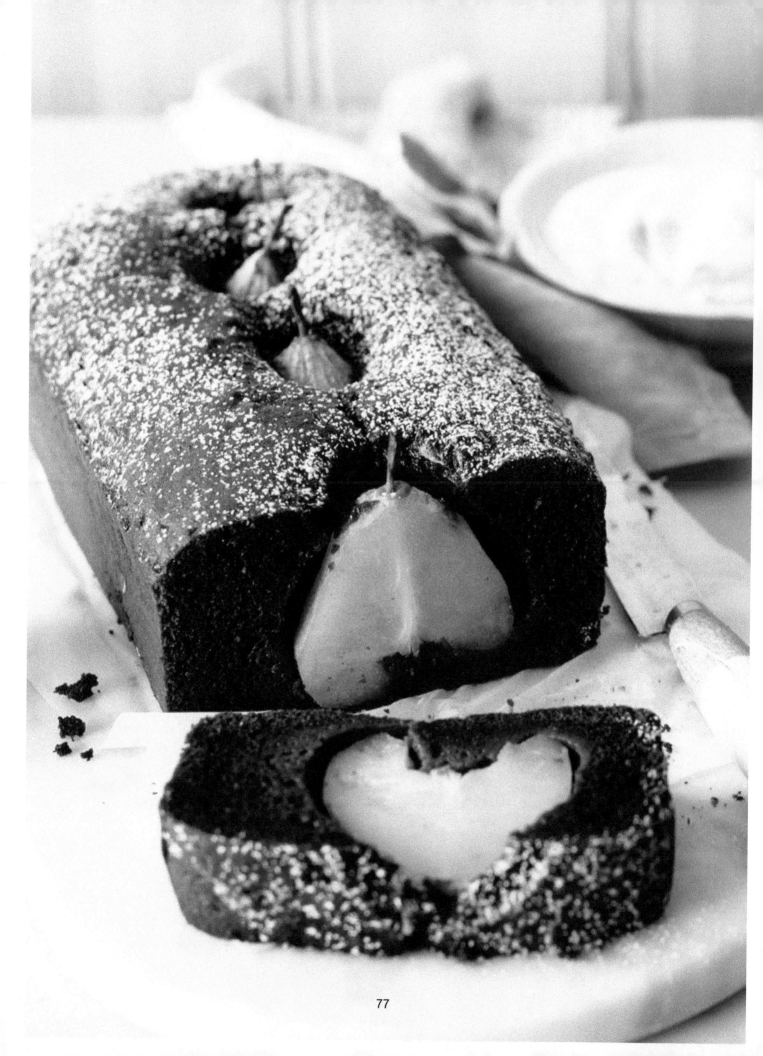

CHOCOLATE
pear loaf

 PREP 15 MINS **COOK** 1 HOUR 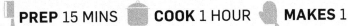 **MAKES** 1

INGREDIENTS

540g Devil's Food cake mix

3 eggs

¾ cup water

⅓ cup vegetable oil

4 medium pears, core removed from base

2 tablespoons icing sugar

METHOD

1. Preheat oven to 180°C. Grease and line a 27cm x 11.5cm x 6.5cm deep (base measurement) (8 cup capacity) loaf pan with baking paper. Prepare cake mix as per packet instructions. Spoon one-third of cake batter into the base of prepared loaf pan. Stand pears in cake batter. Spoon remaining cake batter around and over pears until covered

2. Bake loaf for 50-60 minutes or until cooked through when tested in the centre with a skewer. Allow to stand for 10 minutes before transferring loaf to a wire rack to cool. Dust with icing sugar and serve

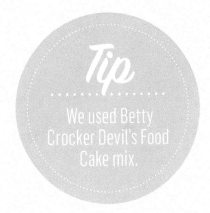

Tip

We used Betty Crocker Devil's Food Cake mix.

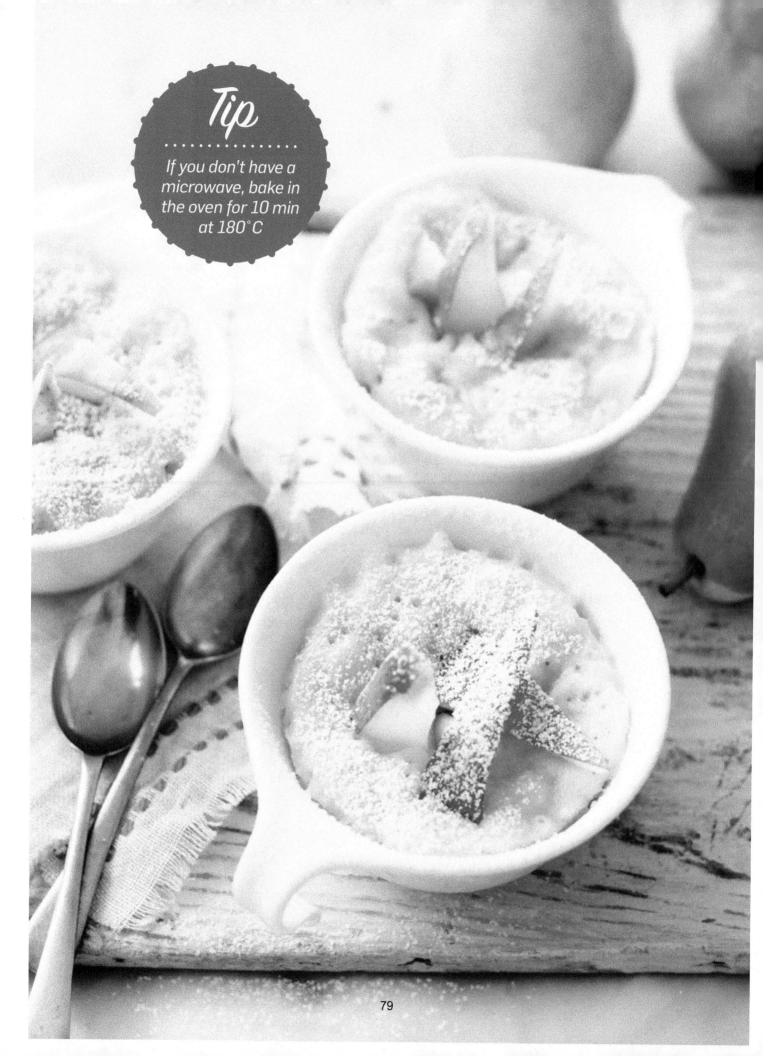

PEAR AND ALMOND
mug cake

 PREP 10 MINS   **COOK** 1 MIN   **SERVES** 4

INGREDIENTS

1 large pear

⅔ cup self-raising flour

2 tablespoons almond meal

2 tablespoons caster sugar

2 eggs

⅓ cup milk

40g butter, melted and cooled

½ teaspoon vanilla

¼ cup maple syrup, to serve

Icing sugar, to dust

METHOD

1. Finely dice half the pear and cut remaining half into thin wedges. Combine flour, almond meal and sugar in a small bowl. Whisk egg, milk, butter and vanilla in a jug. Add to flour mixture and stir until combined. Stir through diced pear

2. Spoon cake batter into 4 x ¾ cup capacity cups. Microwave on high for 60-70 seconds or until cake has risen and top is just set. Stand pear wedges up in cooked cakes. Drizzle with maple syrup and dust with icing sugar. Serve immediately

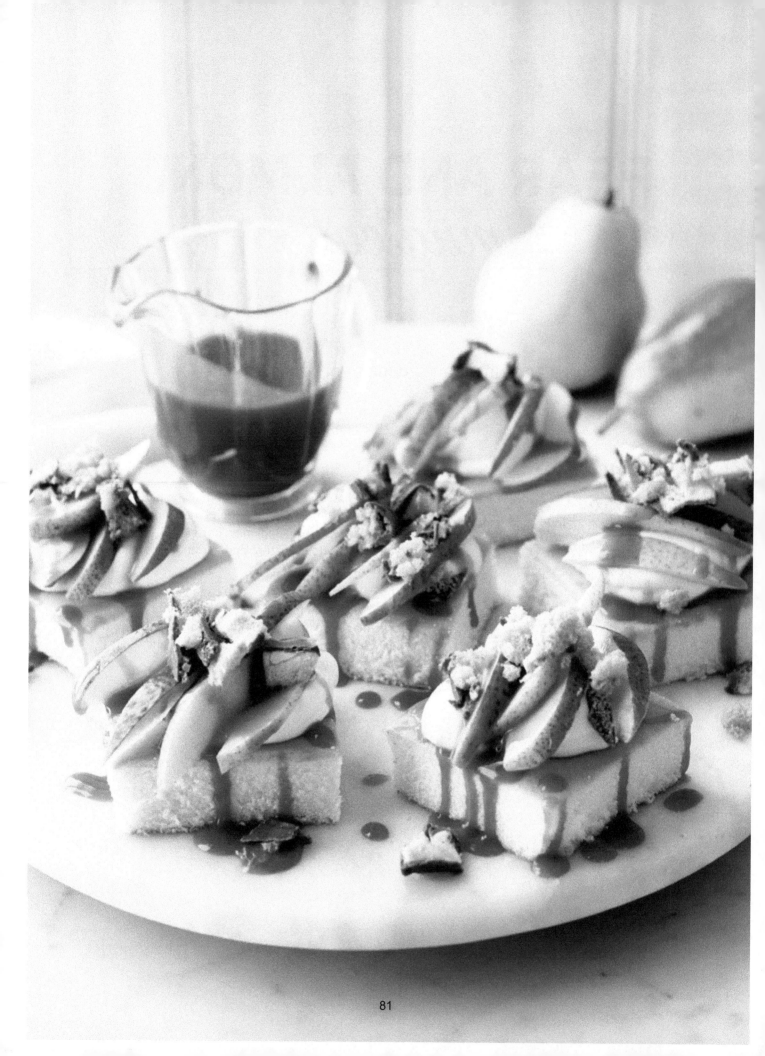

MINI SPONGE CAKES WITH PEARS AND *salted caramel sauce*

 PREP 10 MINS   👤 **SERVES** 6

INGREDIENTS

225g unfilled rectangular sponge slab

150ml tub double thick cream

2 small pears, quartered, core removed, cut into thin wedges

⅓ cup purchased salted caramel flavoured topping

50g hokey pokey honeycomb bar, finely chopped

METHOD

1. Cut sponge slab into 6 squares or using a biscuit cutter, cut into 7cm rounds. Place sponge cake onto serving plates. Top with cream and pear wedges. Drizzle over caramel topping and sprinkle with hokey pokey. Serve

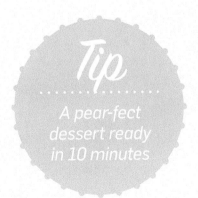

Tip

A pear-fect dessert ready in 10 minutes

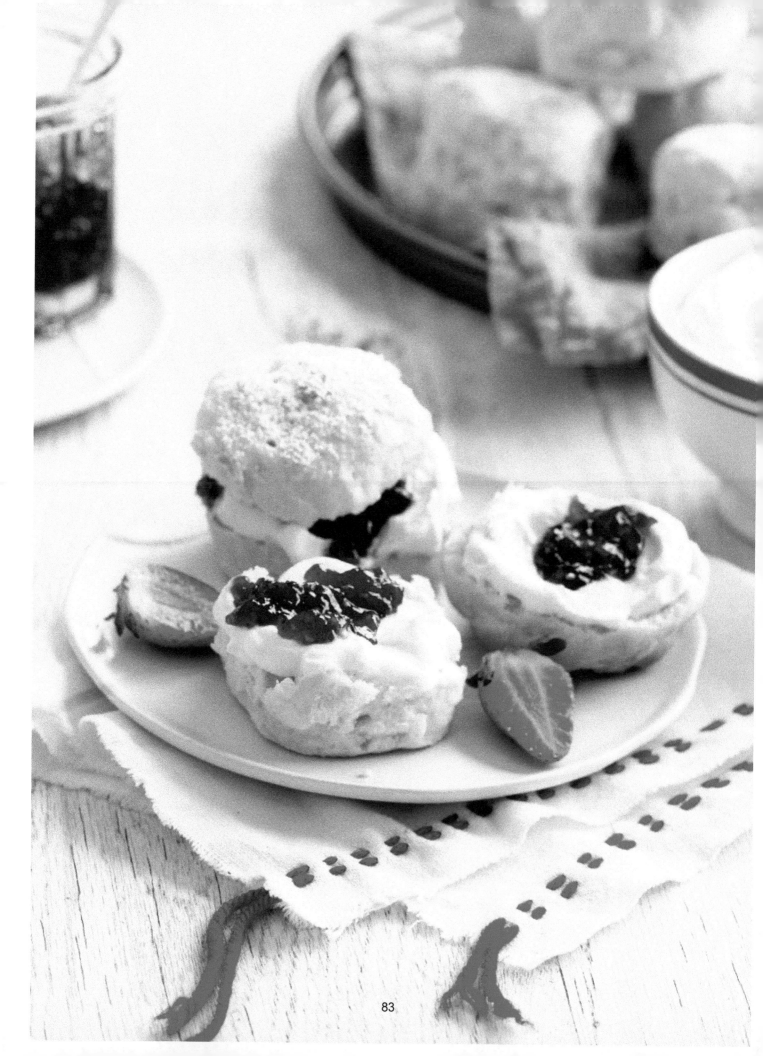

BUTTERMILK & VANILLA BEAN
scones

 PREP 20 MINS   **COOK** 20-23 MINS   **MAKES** 12

INGREDIENTS

3 cups self-raising flour

2 teaspoons baking powder

½ teaspoon salt

¼ cup caster sugar

4 tablespoons (80 g) Western Star Spreadable Original Soft, chilled

1½ cups buttermilk (plus extra for brushing)

1 teaspoon vanilla bean paste or extract

Icing sugar, for dusting

300 mL Western Star Thickened Cream, whipped, and raspberry jam, to serve

METHOD

1. Preheat oven to 220°C/200°C fan-forced. Place flour, baking powder, salt and sugar into a large bowl. Dot with the Western Star Spreadable Original Soft. Using your fingertips, rub together until mixture resembles fine breadcrumbs

2. Make a well in the centre of the dry ingredients. Whisk buttermilk and vanilla in a jug. Pour mixture into dry ingredients. Using a dinner knife, quickly mix until just combined (add a little more buttermilk to the mixture if needed). Pull dough together into a rough ball. Turn onto a lightly floured surface and gently knead just until a smooth dough forms. Press the dough into a 3 cm thick circle. Using a 5 cm cookie cutter dusted with flour, cut 12 rounds from the dough (re-rolling dough as necessary)

3. Place scones close together onto a lightly greased baking tray lined with baking paper. Brush tops with extra buttermilk. Bake for 20-23 minutes until pale golden and cooked through. Remove scones from pan and wrap in a clean tea-towel. Set aside to cool slightly

4. Dust warm scones with icing sugar. Serve split scones topped with whipped cream and raspberry jam. Add fresh seasonal berries, if liked

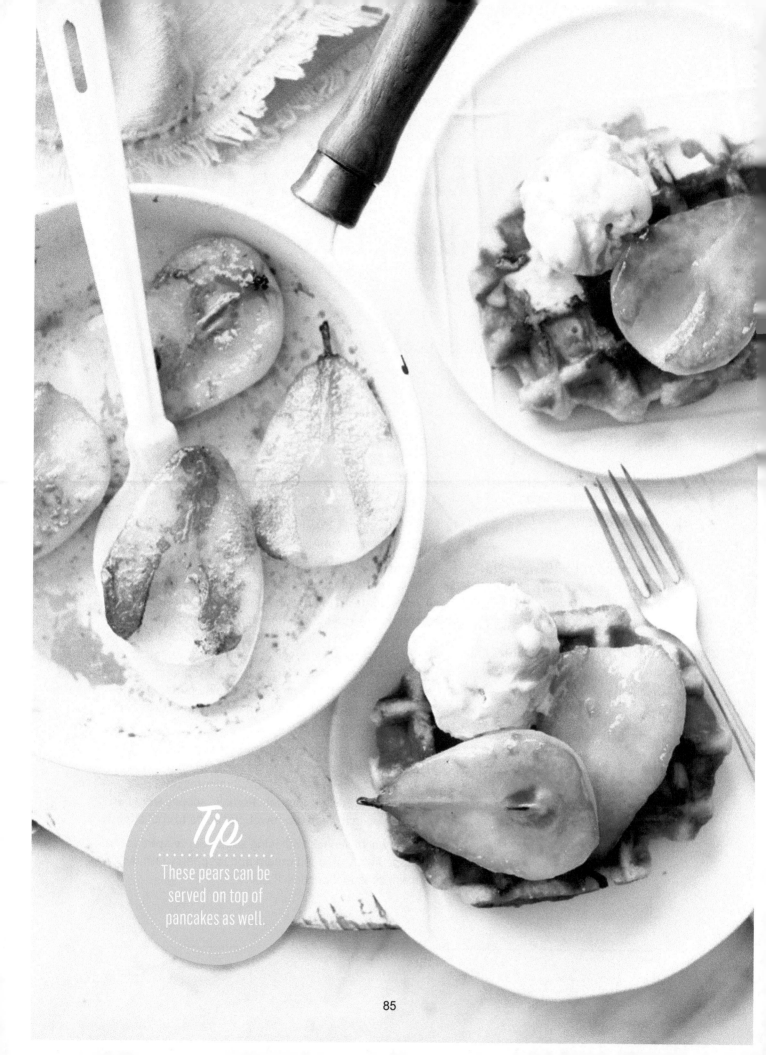

Tip

These pears can be served on top of pancakes as well.

WAFFLES WITH CARAMEL ICE CREAM
and pears

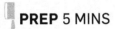 **PREP** 5 MINS **COOK** 10 MINS 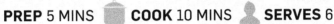 **SERVES** 6

INGREDIENTS

25g butter

2 tablespoon brown sugar

6 small pears, peeled, halved

6 thick waffles

Salted caramel ice cream, to serve

METHOD

1. Melt butter in a frying pan over medium heat. When sizzling add the brown sugar and stir until sugar has melted. Add pears, cut side down and cook for 3 minutes. Turn and cook for 3 minutes or until pears are caramelised and softened. Remove from heat and cool

2. Toast waffles and place onto serving plates. Top with a small scoop of ice cream. Place pear and sauce over ice cream and serve immediately

BABIES
6-9 MONTHS

Sweet potatoes are the perfect veg for mashing and blending into delicious purees for little ones.

TIP

Parsnip will take the longest to cook, so once that is tender the rest will be too.

SWEET POTATO & ROAST VEGETABLE PUREE

Prep Time: 10 minutes
Cook Time: 40 minutes
Makes: approx 2 ½ cups

Ingredients

350g Sweet Potato

1 large carrot (180g)

1 large zucchini (150g)

1 small parsnip (120g)

1 tablespoon olive oil

Method

1. Preheat oven to 220°C/200°C fan-forced. Line an oven tray with baking paper

2. Peel sweet potato and carrot and coarsely chop all vegetables (about 2cm pieces). Place on tray and drizzle with oil; tossing to coat

3. Bake for 35-40 min until tender. Transfer to a bowl and add ¾ cup (185ml) - 1 cup (250ml) fresh boiled water. Puree with a stick blender until smooth

SWEET POTATO, BROCCOLI & ZUCCHINI MASH

Prep Time: 10 minutes
Cook Time: 20 minutes
Makes: 3 ½ cups

Ingredients

2 teaspoons olive oil
350g Sweet Potato, chopped
1 potato (200g), chopped
1 small parsnip (120g), chopped
1 large zucchini (150g), chopped
100g small broccoli florets

Method

1. Heat oil in a medium saucepan on high. Add sweet potato, potato and parsnip. Cook, stirring for 2 min. Add ½ cup water. Bring to the boil and simmer for 10 min

2. Add zucchini and broccoli. Stir well and simmer, covered, for a further 10 min until vegetables are tender. Remove from heat and mash to desired consistency

SWEET POTATO & LENTIL PUREE

Prep Time: 10 minutes
Cook Time: 20 minutes
Makes: 2 ¼ cups

Ingredients

1 tablespoon olive oil
1 small onion (80g), chopped
1 large carrot (180g), peeled, chopped
½ teaspoon ground cumin
300g Sweet Potato, peeled, chopped
½ cup (100g) red lentils, rinsed

Method

1. Heat oil in a saucepan over medium-high heat. Sauté onion for 3-4 min until tender. Add carrot, cook, stirring for 2 min. Add in cumin and cook until fragrant

2. Add sweet potato, lentils and 2 cups (500ml) water. Bring to the boil and simmer, covered for 15-20 min until lentils and vegetables are tender

3. Remove from heat; cool slightly. Puree with a stick blender until smooth

BABY-LED WEANING

9-12 MONTHS

If your baby is eager to begin feeding themselves, it may be time to push away those purees and serve them up some soft sweet potato bites.

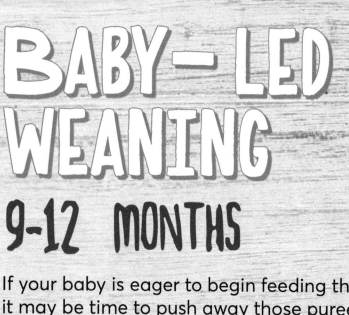

SWEET POTATO, CHEESE & BACON PIZZAS

Prep Time: 5 minutes
Cook Time: 15 minutes
Makes: 6

Ingredients

250g Sweet Potato, unpeeled, sliced into 5mm slices

Spray oil

2 tablespoons tomato paste

60g shaved ham, chopped

½ cup grated mozzarella cheese

Baby basil leaves, to serve

Method

1. Preheat oven to 220°C/200°C fan-forced. Line an oven tray with baking paper

2. Place sweet potato rounds on tray. Spray with oil. Bake for 10 min until almost just tender

3. Spread rounds with tomato paste. Top with ham and cheese. Grill for 3-4 min until golden. Serve topped with basil leaves

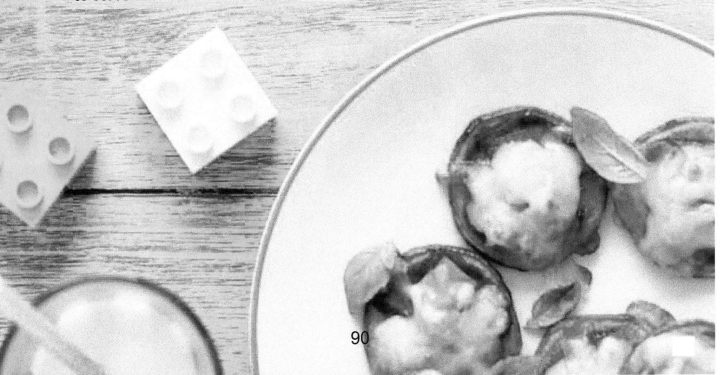

90

LAMB CUTLETS WITH SWEET POTATO & PEARL COUSCOUS

Prep Time: 10 minutes
Cook Time: 15 minutes
Makes: 4

Ingredients

250g Sweet Potato, peeled, cut into 2cm cubes

2 teaspoons olive oil, plus extra for lamb

125g (⅔ cup) pearl couscous

1 cup salt reduced chicken stock or water

1 sprig rosemary

4 lamb cutlets

Pinch mild paprika

Method

1. Microwave, steam or boil sweet potato until tender. Set aside

2. Meanwhile, heat oil in a medium saucepan over medium-high heat. Add couscous and cook, stirring, for 3 min until couscous is golden. Add stock and rosemary. Bring to the boil. Reduce heat and simmer, covered for 10 min or until couscous is tender

3. Set aside for 5 min or until liquid is absorbed. Use a fork to separate grains. Add sweet potato and set aside

4. Meanwhile, drizzle a little olive oil over lamb, Sprinkle with paprika. Heat oil in a large frying pan on high. Cook lamb for 2-3 min each side until cooked to taste. Set aside to rest for 5 min. Serve with couscous

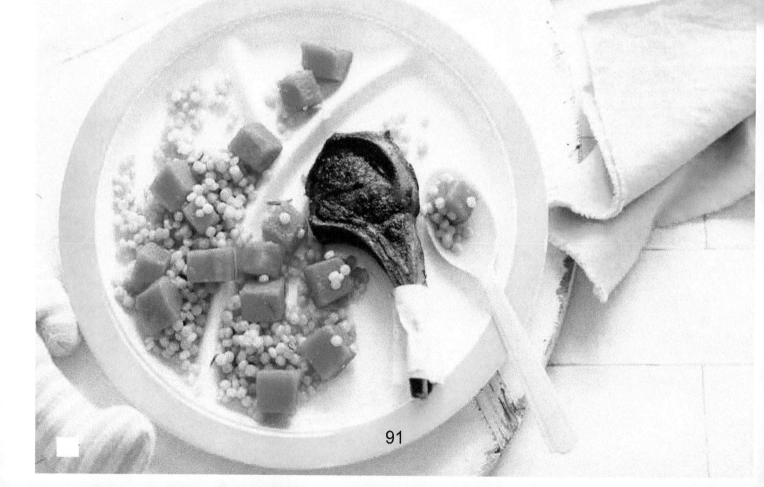

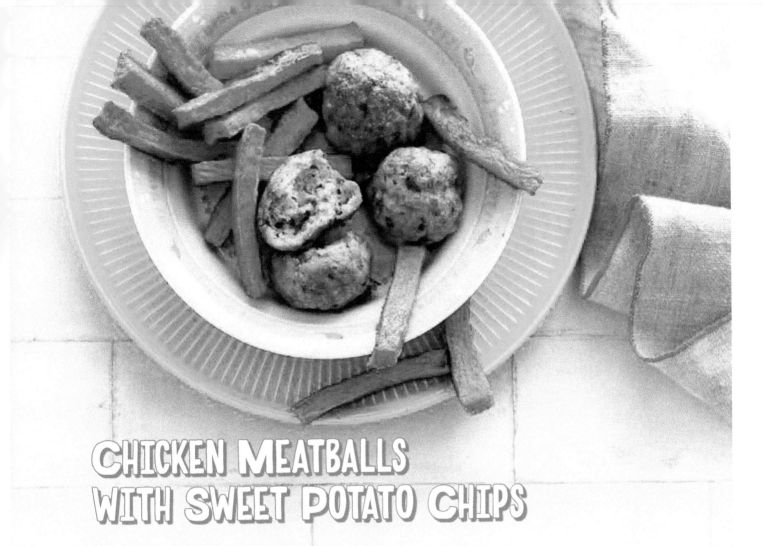

CHICKEN MEATBALLS WITH SWEET POTATO CHIPS

Prep Time: 20 minutes
Cook Time: 1 hour
Makes: 4

Ingredients

CHICKEN MEATBALLS

500g chicken mince

1 cup breadcrumbs

1 egg

⅓ cup finely grated parmesan

2 tablespoons finely chopped flat-leaf parsley

SWEET POTATO CHIPS

350g Sweet Potato, peeled, cut into chips

2 teaspoons olive oil

Pinch paprika

Method

CHICKEN MEATBALLS

1. Preheat oven to 220°C/200°C fan-forced. Line 2 oven trays with baking paper

2. Combine mince, breadcrumbs, egg, parmesan and parsley in a bowl. Roll heaped tablespoons of mixture into balls. Place on one of the trays

3. Bake for 20-25 min until golden and cooked through

SWEET POTATO CHIPS

1. Meanwhile place chips on remaining tray and toss with oil and paprika. Bake for 25-30 min until golden and tender

2. Serve meatballs with chips

92

TODDLER TO SCHOOL AGE

1-12 YEARS

The little ones in your life will love these tasty and wholesome dishes, and so will you.

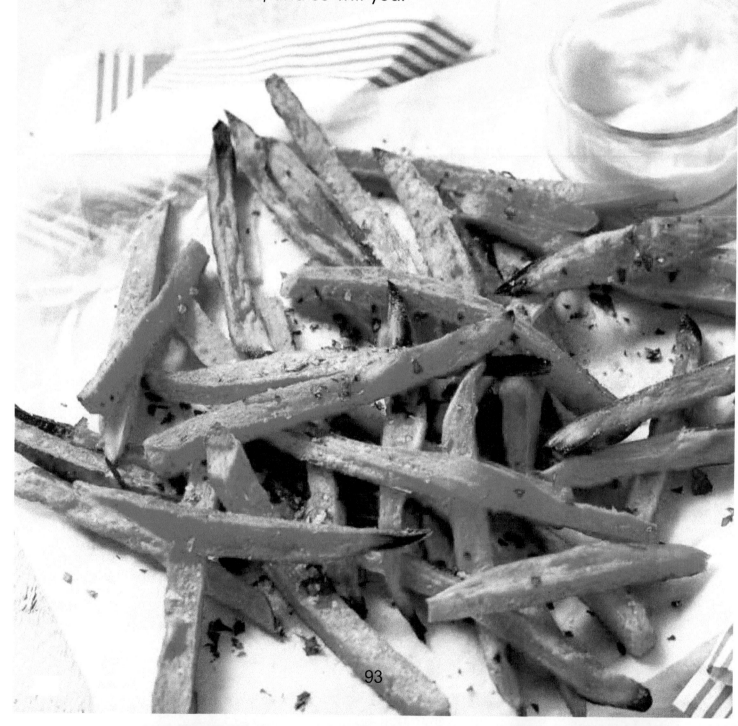

SWEET POTATO FRIES

Prep Time: 10 minutes, plus soaking time
Cook Time: 40 minutes
Serves: 4-6

Ingredients

400g Sweet Potato, peeled, cut into 1cm chips

2 teaspoons corn flour

Pinch mild paprika

Spray oil

Natural yoghurt, to serve

Method

1. Soak chips in water for 1 hour to remove starch. Drain and pat-dry on paper towel

2. Meanwhile, preheat oven to 220°C /200°C fan-forced. Line 2 trays with baking paper

3. Place chips in zip-lock bag with corn flour and paprika. Shake well until evenly coated

4. Place chips in a single layer on trays. Spray with oil and bake for 25-30 minutes, turning once. Season to taste. Serve with yoghurt

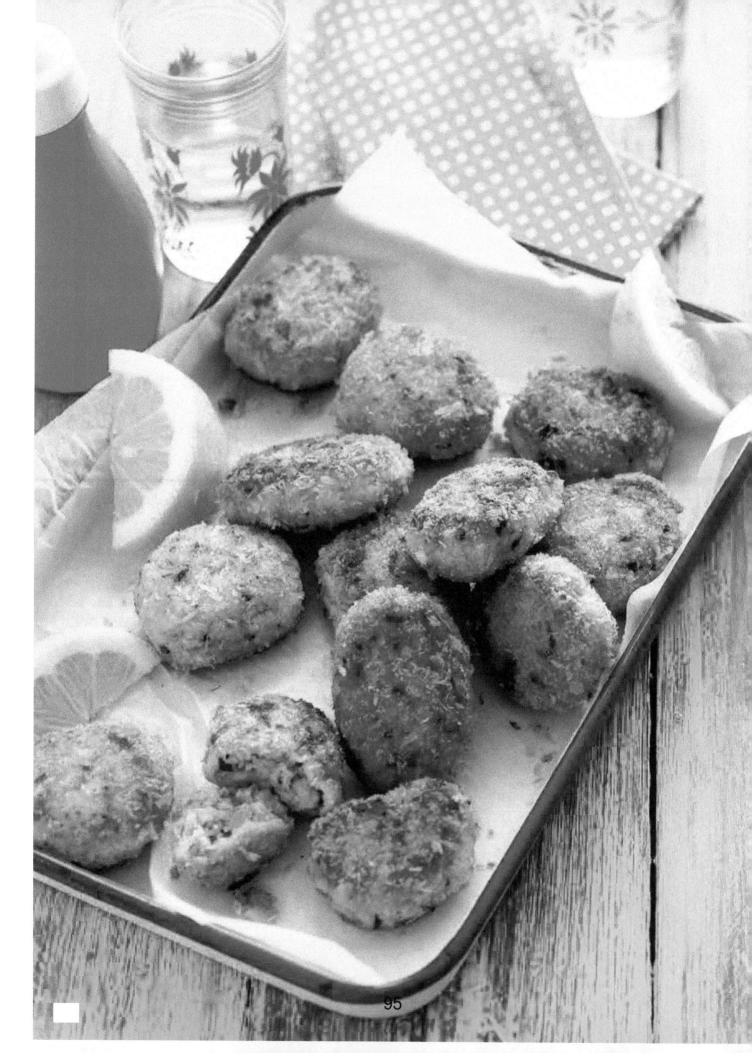

SWEET POTATO, CHICKEN AND COUSCOUS NUGGETS

Prep Time: 25 minutes
Cook Time: 25 minutes
Makes: 35

Ingredients

½ cup couscous

½ cup Sweet Potato puree*

2 teaspoons olive oil

1 small brown onion, finely chopped

500g chicken mince

1 small apple, peeled, cored, coarsely grated

1 egg

1 tablespoon chopped parsley

1 cup panko breadcrumbs

Oil, for shallow frying

Method

1. Place couscous in a heatproof bowl. Cover with ½ cup boiling water. Cover and stand for 5 minutes; separate grains with a fork. Cool

2. Meanwhile, heat oil in a large frying pan on high. Sauté onion for 4-5 minutes until very tender. Transfer to a large bowl. Cool

3. Add couscous, mince, apple, sweet potato puree, egg and parsley in a bowl. Season to taste. Roll tablespoons of mixture into balls. Flatten slightly and coat in breadcrumbs

4. Heat oil in same pan, cook nuggets for 2-3 minutes, each side until golden and cooked through. Drain on paper towel

Tips

*Microwave cubed Sweet Potato until soft (1-2 mins), then mash with a fork.

Uncooked mixture can be frozen. Defrost in the fridge before rolling into nuggets and crumbing

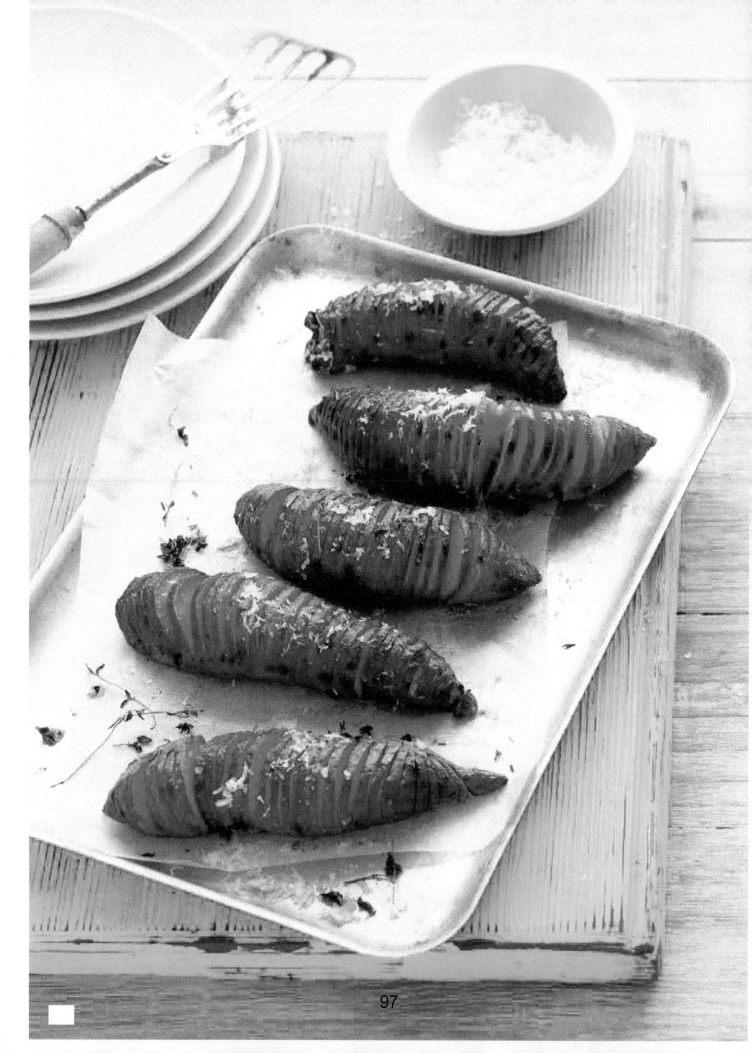

HASSELBACK SWEET POTATOES

Prep Time: 15 minutes

Cook Time: 1 hour 10 minutes

Serves: 6

Ingredients

6 x 200g Sweet Potatoes, scrubbed

6 sprigs fresh thyme, plus extra for serving

olive oil

¼ teaspoon sea salt

⅓ cup finely grated parmesan

Method

1. Preheat oven to 200°C/180°C fan-forced. Carefully cut 3mm slices into the sweet potatoes, leaving 5mm intact at the bottom. Place on a baking-paper lined oven tray

2. Strip the leaves from the thyme and tuck in between the fans of the sweet potatoes

3. Drizzle with olive oil and sprinkle with salt and pepper

4. Bake for 1 hour - 1 hour 10 minutes until golden and soft in the middle when easily pierced with a knife. Serve sprinkled with parmesan

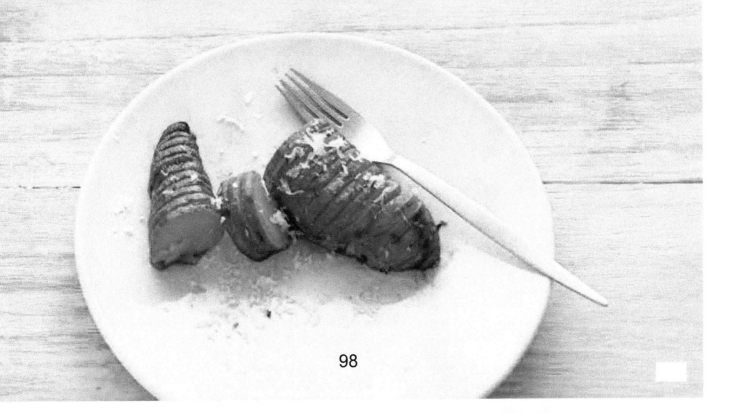

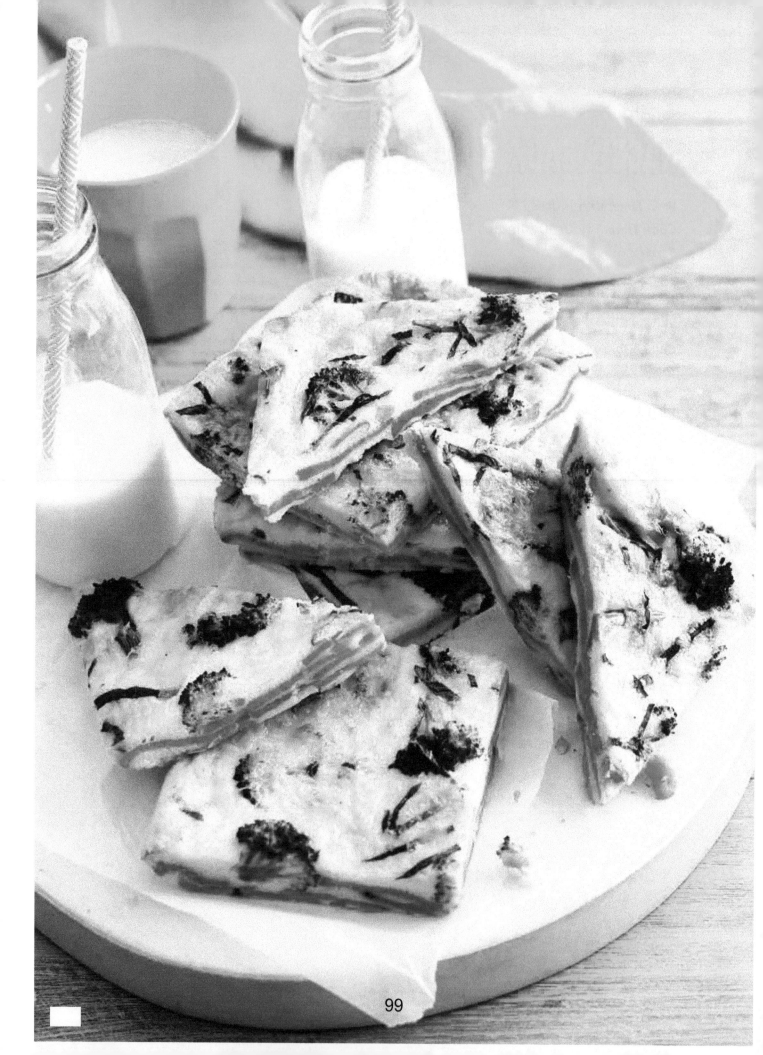

SWEET POTATO AND BROCCOLI FRITTATA

Prep Time: 20 minutes
Cook Time: 50 minutes
Serves: 6

Ingredients

500g Sweet Potato, peeled, thinly sliced

Olive oil spray

8 eggs

½ cup (125ml) light thickened cream

¾ cup (90g) grated tasty cheese

100g small broccoli florets, blanched

2 tablespoons shredded basil

Method

1. Preheat oven to 200°C/180°C fan-forced. Lightly grease and line base and sides of a 20 x 30cm rectangular slice pan

2. Place sweet potato on a lined oven tray. Spray with oil and bake for 15-20 minutes until tender

3. Beat eggs, cream and half of the cheese together. Layer sweet potato and broccoli over base of pan. Pour over egg mixture. Sprinkle with basil and remaining cheese

4. Bake for 25-30 minutes until golden and set. Stand for 5 minutes before slicing

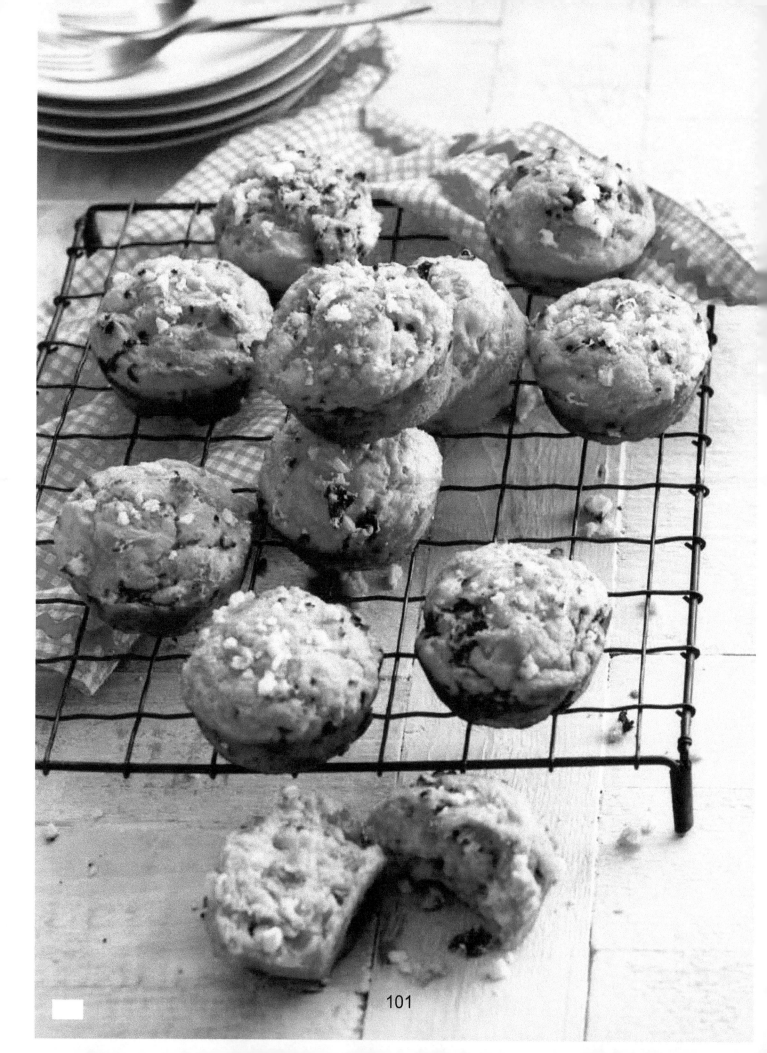

SWEET POTATO, SPINACH AND FETA MUFFINS

Prep Time: 30 minutes
Cook Time: 30 minutes
Makes: 12

Ingredients

1 cup (150g) plain flour

1 cup (160g) wholemeal plain flour

1 teaspoon bi-carb soda

40g baby spinach leaves, steamed, chopped

2 green onions, sliced thinly

100g feta, crumbled

2 eggs, beaten

⅔ cup (190g) plain Greek style yoghurt

125g can creamed corn

1 cup Sweet Potato puree

50g butter, melted

¼ cup (20g) grated parmesan

Method

1. Preheat oven to 200°C/180°C fan-forced. Lightly grease a 12-hole muffin pan

2. Sift flour and soda together in a large bowl. Stir in spinach, onion and half of the feta. Combine remaining ingredients in a bowl, whisking well to combine

3. Fold through dry mixture until just combined. Spoon into prepared cases and sprinkle with remaining feta. Bake for 25-30 minutes until cooked when tested with a skewer

Tips

You will need a 550g Sweet Potato to make enough puree for this recipe.

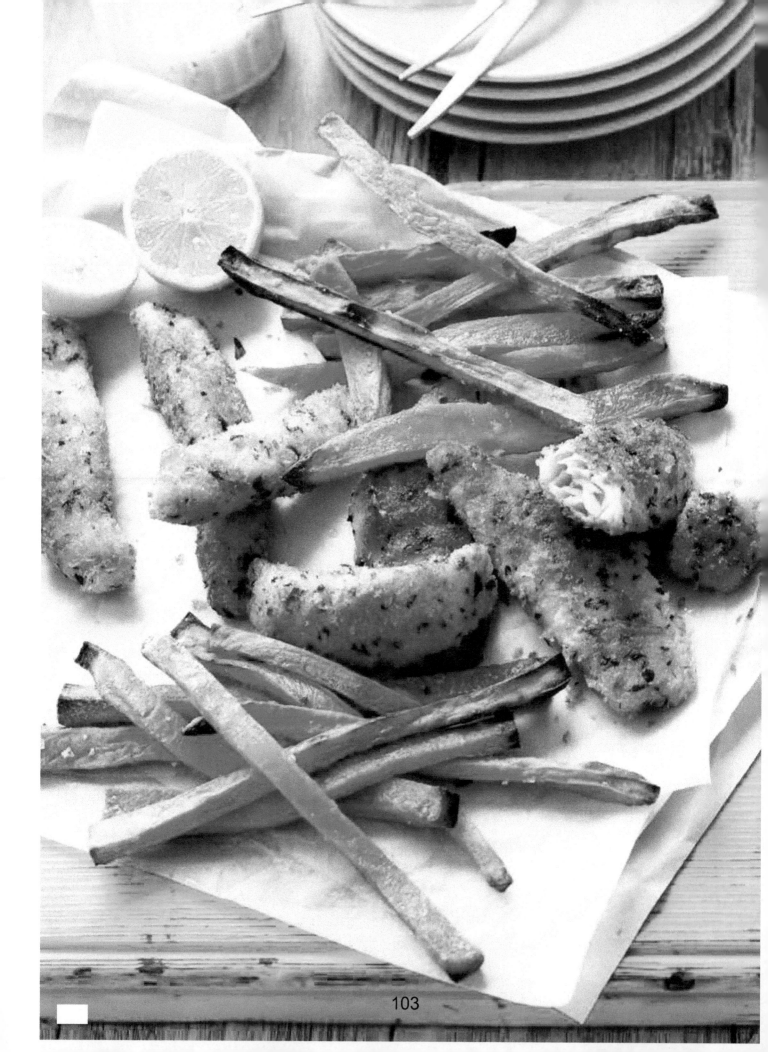

SWEET POTATO FRIES WITH CRUMBED FISH

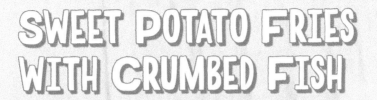

Prep Time: 30 minutes, plus soaking time
Cook Time: 55 minutes
Serves: 4

Ingredients

SWEET POTATO FRIES

400g Sweet Potato, peeled, cut into 1cm chips

2 teaspoons corn flour

Pinch mild paprika

Spray oil

CRUMBED FISH

500g flathead fillets, bones removed, halved

1 egg, beaten lightly

1 cup panko breadcrumbs

1 tablespoon finely chopped flat-leaf parsley

Oil, for shallow frying

Tartar sauce and lemon wedges, to serve

Method

SWEET POTATO FRIES

1. Soak chips in water for 1 hour to remove starch. Drain and pat-dry on paper towel

2. Meanwhile, preheat oven to 220°C /200°C fan-forced. Line 2 trays with baking paper

3. Place chips in zip-lock bag with corn flour and paprika. Shake well until evenly coated

4. Place chips in a single layer on trays. Spray with oil and bake for 25-30 minutes, turning once. Season to taste

CRUMBED FISH

1. Dip fish in egg, shaking off excess. Toss in combined crumb and parsley mixture to coat. Place on a plate

2. Pour enough oil into a large frying pan to come 1cm up side of pan. Heat over medium-high heat. Cook fish, in 3 batches, for 2 minutes each side until golden and cooked through. Drain on paper towel

3. Serve fish with sweet potato chips and tartar sauce

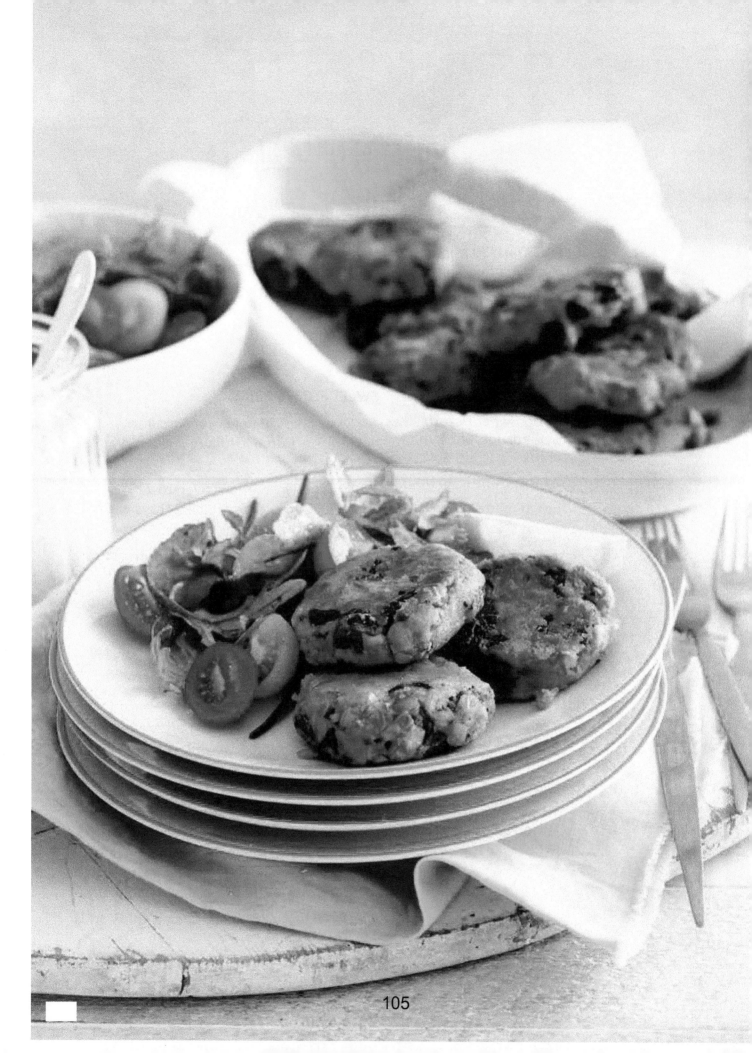

SWEET POTATO AND LENTIL PATTIES

Prep Time: 25 minutes
Cook Time: 30 minutes
Makes: 12

Ingredients

½ cup brown lentils

500g Sweet Potato, peeled, cubed

2 tablespoons olive oil

1 small onion, finely chopped

2 garlic cloves, crushed

1 teaspoon ground cumin

½ teaspoon ground coriander

½ teaspoon turmeric

60g baby spinach, roughly chopped

⅓ cup plain flour

Natural yoghurt and lemon wedges, to serve

Method

1. Preheat oven to 220°C /200°C fan-forced. Line an oven tray with baking paper. Place sweet potato on tray and drizzle with half of the oil. Bake for 15-20 minutes until tender. Mash in a bowl and set aside

2. Cook lentils in a pan of boiling water for 15-20 minutes until softened. Drain well. Transfer to a large bowl to cool

3. Meanwhile, heat oil in a large frying pan on medium. Cook onion and garlic for 4-5 minutes until softened. Add spices and cook for 1 minute until fragrant. Add spinach, stirring until just wilted. Transfer to bowl with lentils and sweet potato. Mix well and season to taste. Chill until cold. Form into patties and toss in flour to coat. Place on a baking paper-lined tray

4. Heat oil in frying pan on medium-high. Cook patties for 2-3 minutes each side until golden. Drain on paper towel. Serve patties with yoghurt and lemon wedges

Tips

Brown lentils are also labelled as green lentils. They are larger than the French lentils.

For gluten free option – replace plain flour for gluten-free flour.

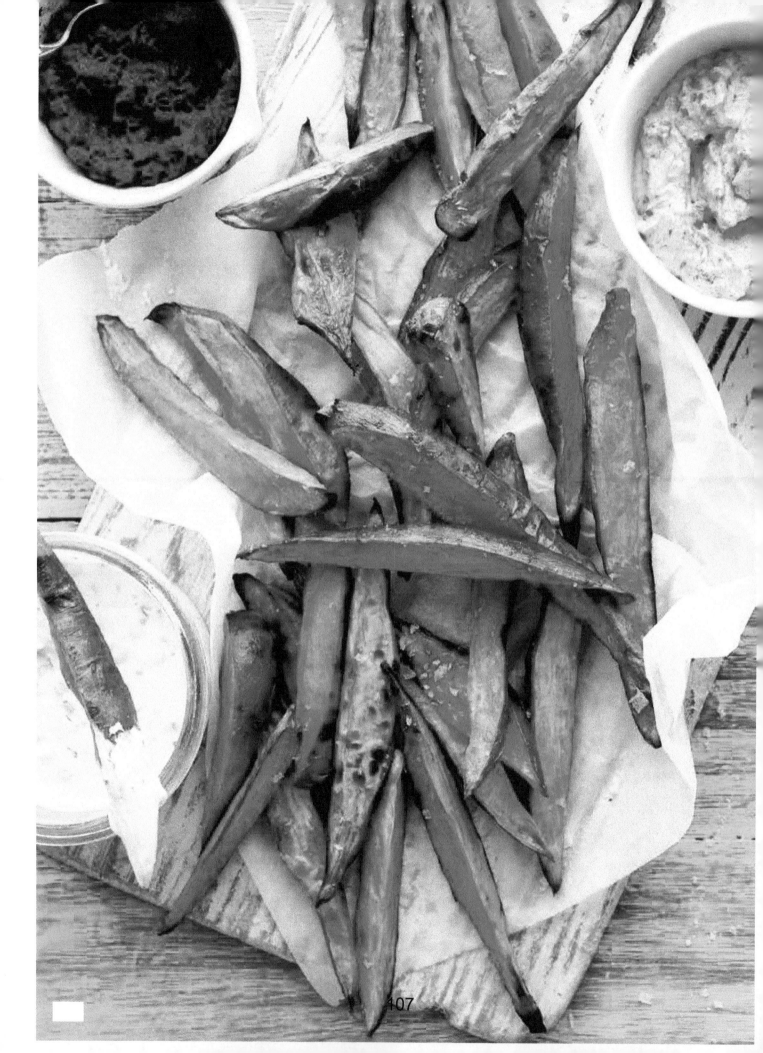

SWEET POTATO WEDGES WITH DIPS

Prep Time: 10 minutes
Cook Time: 40 minutes
Serves: 6

Ingredients

3 small Sweet Potatoes (about 600g), scrubbed cut into wedges

2 tablespoons olive oil

Beetroot dip, semi-dried tomato dip, tzatziki, to serve

Method

1. Preheat oven to 220°C/200°C fan forced. Line 2 oven trays with baking paper

2. Arrange wedges on trays, leaving a space between each one. Drizzle with olive oil and bake about 30-35 minutes, turning once. Season to taste and serve with dips

Tips

Use any selection of dips of choice.

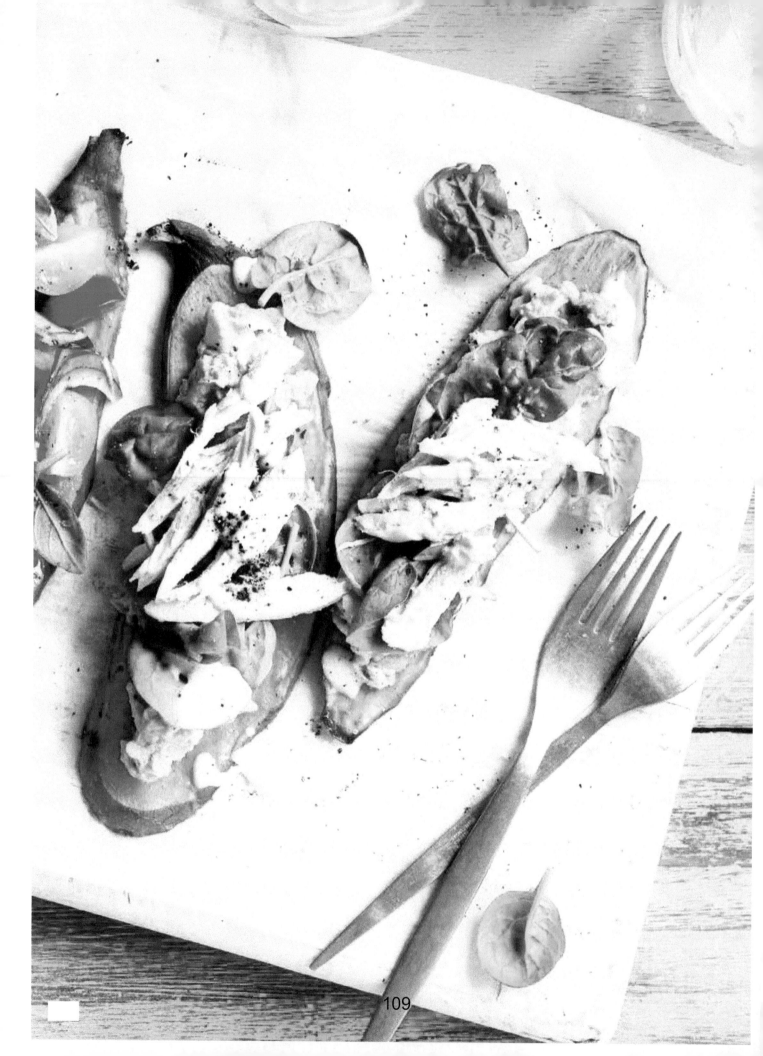

SWEET POTATO TOAST TOPPED WITH MASHED AVOCADO, CHICKEN AND AIOLI

Prep Time: 15 minutes
Cook Time: 15 minutes
Serves: 6

Ingredients

6 slices (5mm thick) Sweet Potato, skin on

1 avocado, mashed

¾ cup baby spinach leaves

1 cup shredded BBQ chicken

¼ cup aioli

Method

1. Preheat oven to 200°C /180°C fan-forced. Line an oven tray with baking paper. Arrange slices on tray. Spray with oil and season to taste. Bake for 10-15 minutes until golden and tender

2. Spread toasts with avocado. Top with spinach and chicken. Drizzle with aioli. Serve immediately

Tips

You can also cook toasts in a sandwich press (between 2 sheets of baking paper) for about 5 minutes until browned and tender.

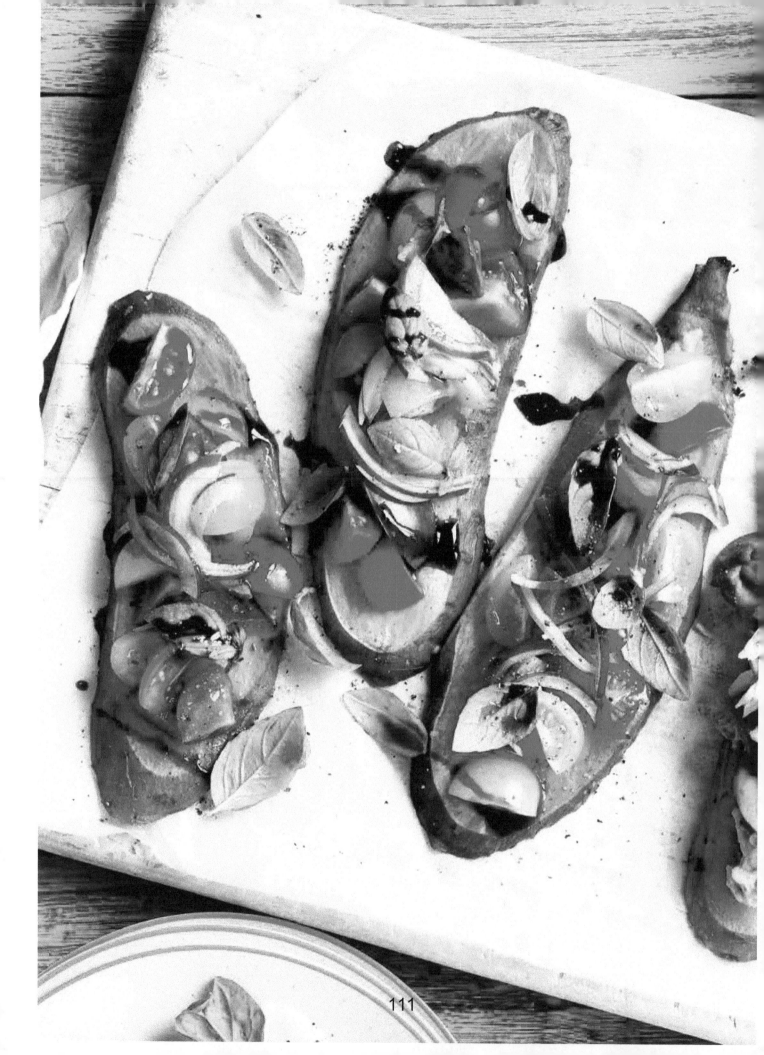

SWEET POTATO TOAST TOPPED WITH TOMATO MEDLEY AND BALSAMIC GLAZE

Prep Time: 15 minutes
Cook Time: 15 minutes
Serves: 6

Ingredients

6 slices (5mm thick) Sweet Potato, skin on

200g tomato medley, chopped

½ red onion, thinly sliced

Baby basil leaves and balsamic glaze, to serve

Method

1. Preheat oven to 200°C /180°C fan-forced. Line an oven tray with baking paper. Arrange slices on tray. Spray with oil and season to taste. Bake for 10-15 minutes until golden and tender

2. Top toasts with tomatoes and onion. Sprinkle with basil leaves and drizzle with balsamic glaze. Serve immediately

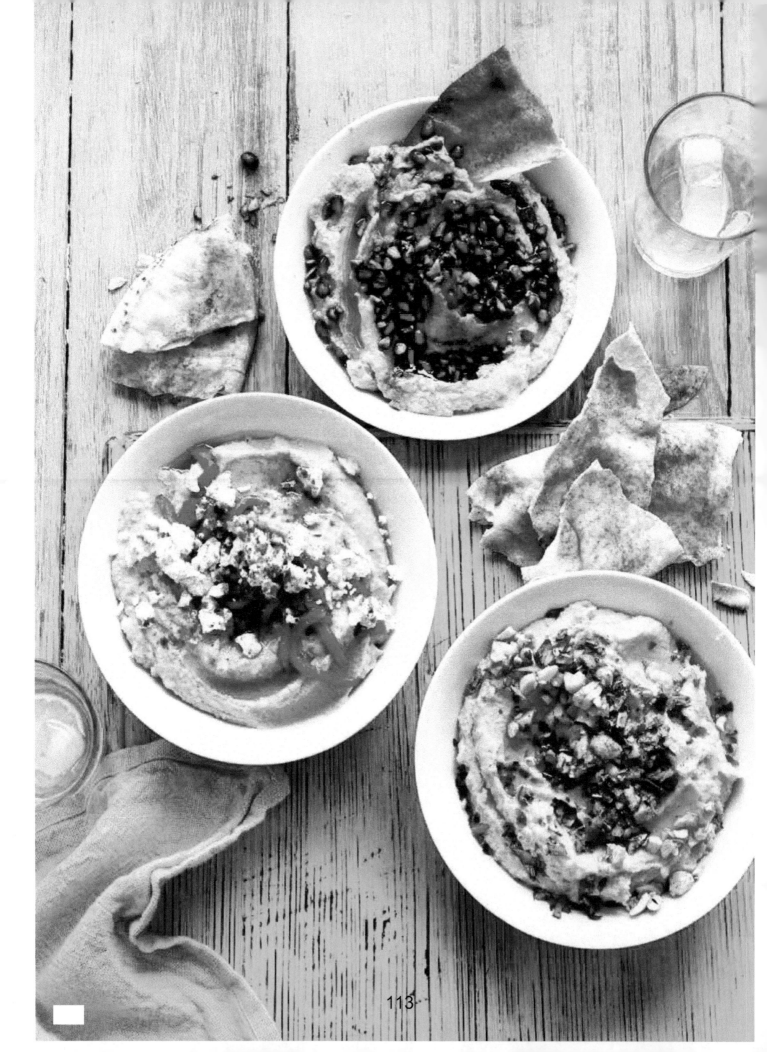

SWEET POTATO HUMMUS – 3 WAYS

BASE RECIPE

Prep Time: 20 minutes
Cook Time: 25 minutes
Makes: 3 cups

Ingredients

400g Sweet Potato, peeled, cubed

1 tablespoon olive oil

400g can chickpeas, rinsed, drained

2 tablespoons tahini

2 tablespoons lemon juice

1 clove garlic, chopped

Olive oil and pita bread crisps, to serve

Method

1. Preheat oven to 200°C /180°C fan-forced. Line an oven tray with baking paper

2. Place sweet potato on tray and drizzle with oil. Toss well and season

3. Bake for 20-25 minutes until tender and golden. Set aside to cool

4. Place sweet potato, chickpeas, tahini, lemon juice and garlic in a food processor. Process with enough warm water until smooth. Season. Serve drizzled with olive oil. Accompany with pita crisps

CORIANDER HUMMUS WITH HONEY ROASTED CASHEWS

Ingredients

2 tablespoons chopped coriander

2 tablespoons chopped honey roasted cashews

1 teaspoon dried chili flakes

Method

1. Top hummus with coriander, cashews and chili flakes. Serve drizzled with olive oil. Accompany with pita crisps

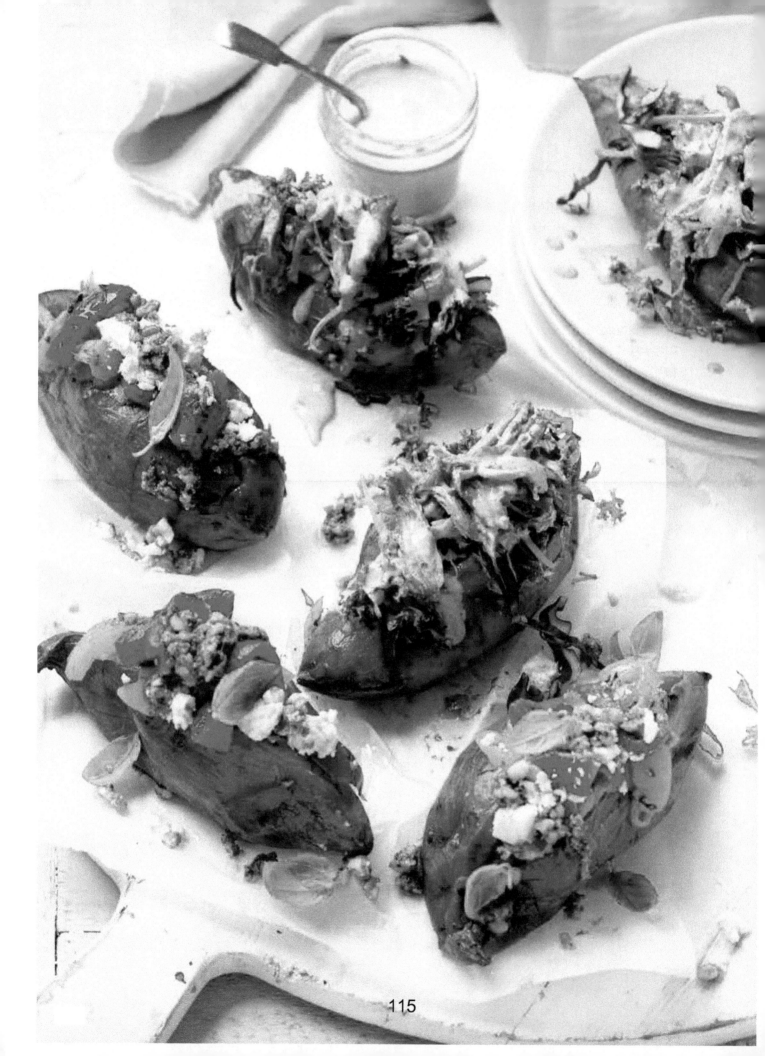

STAND AND STUFF SWEET POTATOES

Prep Time: 20 minutes

Cook Time: 40 minutes

Serves: 4

Ingredients

4 small Sweet Potatoes (about 200g each)

1 tablespoon olive oil

1 cup shredded kale leaves

1 cup shredded red cabbage

1 small carrot, cut into matchsticks

2 green onions, sliced thinly

250g pulled pork

CHIPOTLE AIOLI

½ cup aioli

2 chipotle chillies in abodo sauce

Method

1. Preheat oven to 200°C /180°C fan-forced. Prick sweet potato all over with a small sharp knife. Place two sweet potatoes in a heatproof bowl. Cover with cling film and microwave for 4 minutes. Turn and cook for further 4 minutes. Repeat with remaining sweet potatoes

2. Place sweet potatoes on a lined oven tray. Drizzle with oil and bake for 25-30 minutes until very tender and golden

3. Combine kale, cabbage, carrot and onion in a bowl

4. Split the sweet potatoes down the centre with a sharp knife and ease open. Divide slaw and pork between potatoes. Blend or process aioli and chillies until smooth. Drizzle over pork

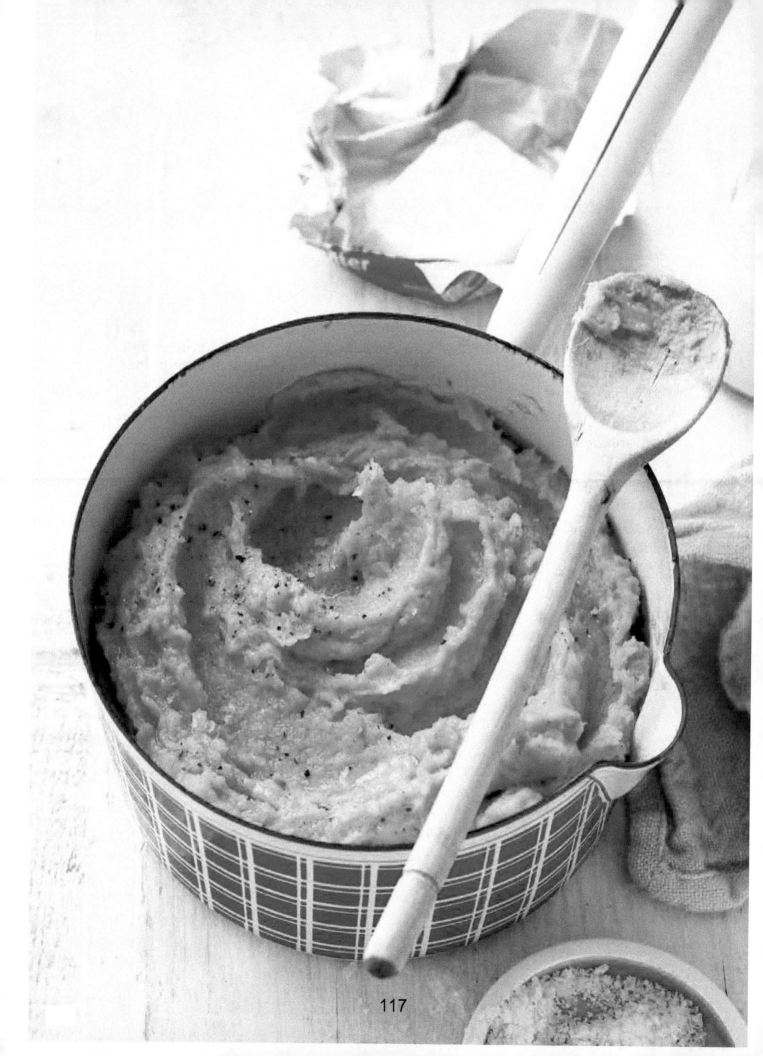

117

ULTIMATE SWEET POTATO MASH

Prep Time: 10 minutes
Cook Time: 15 minutes
Serves: 4

Ingredients

800g Sweet Potato, peeled, chopped

½ cup thickened cream

60g butter

Salt and pepper

Method

1. Place the sweet potatoes in a steaming basket over a medium pan of water and steam for 15 minutes or until tender

2. Place in a large bowl with cream and butter. Mash with a potato masher until smooth. Season with salt and pepper

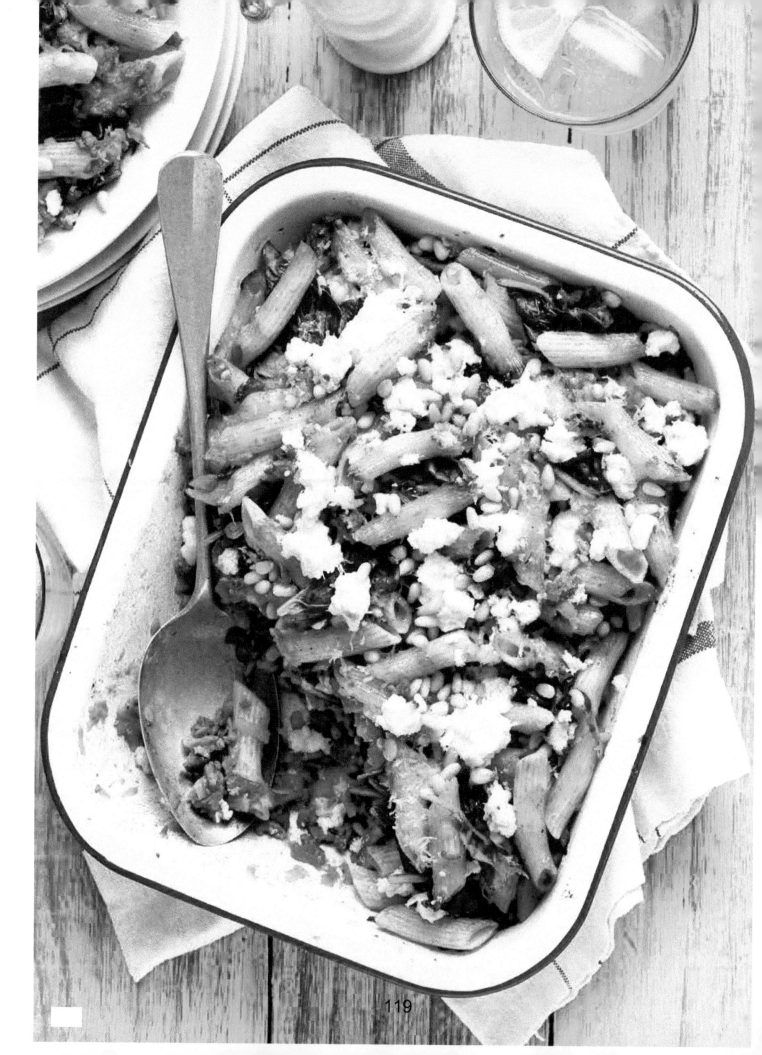

SWEET POTATO PASTA BAKE WITH SPINACH & PINE NUTS

Prep Time: 20 minutes
Cook Time: 50 minutes
Makes: 6

Ingredients

350g penne or other pasta

1 tablespoon olive oil

1 small onion, finely chopped

2 garlic cloves, crushed

500g lean beef mince

400g Sweet Potato, peeled, coarsely grated

1 small zucchini, coarsely grated

2 tablespoons tomato paste

400g can diced tomatoes

1 cup salt-reduced beef stock

4 sprigs thyme

50g baby spinach leaves

100g ricotta

½ cup (40g) grated parmesan

2 tablespoons pine nuts

Method

1. Cook pasta in a large pan of salted, boiling water until al dente. Drain well

2. Meanwhile, heat oil in a medium pan on medium-high heat. Cook onion and garlic for 3-4 min until softened. Add beef and cook until browned, breaking up lumps with a spoon. Add sweet potato and zucchini. Cook for 2 min until softened slightly

3. Add paste, tomatoes, stock and thyme. Simmer, uncovered for 15-20 min until thickened slightly. Stir through spinach leaves until wilted

4. Meanwhile, preheat oven to 220°C/200°C fan-forced

5. Combine pasta and beef mixture in an 8-cup capacity ovenproof dish. Sprinkle with ricotta, parmesan and pine nuts. Bake for 15-20 min until golden

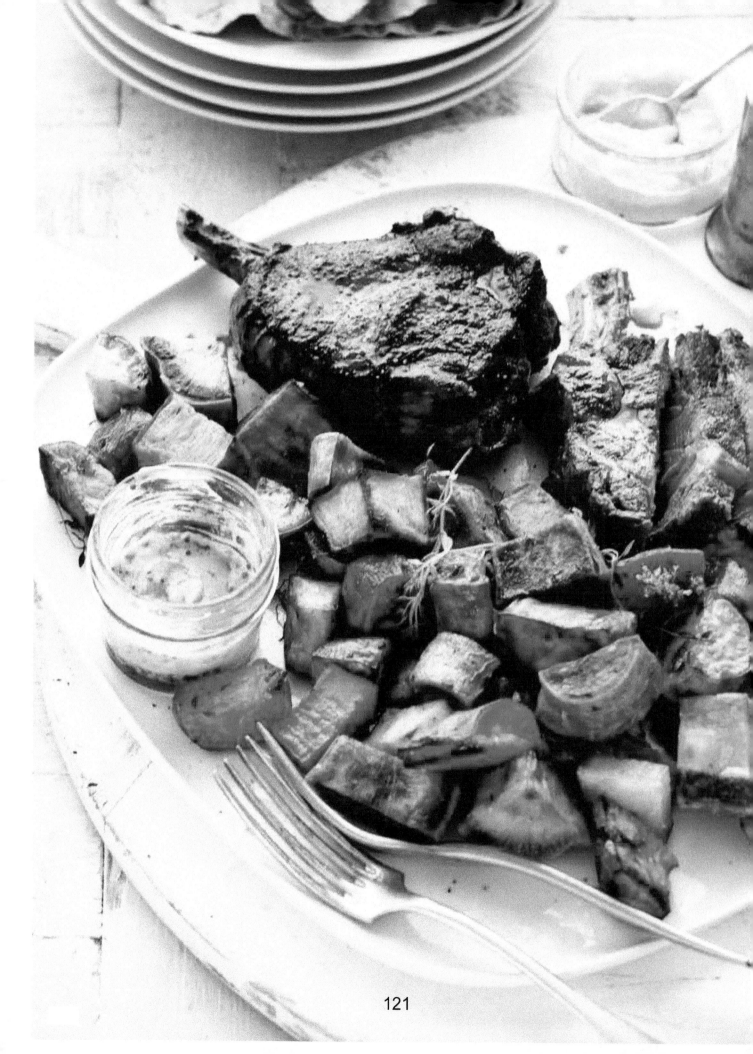

ROAST SWEET POTATO MEDLEY WITH RIB-EYE STEAK

Prep Time: 10 minutes
Cook Time: 50 minutes
Serves: 4

Ingredients

400g each Gold, Purple and White Sweet Potato, chopped

3 tablespoons olive oil, plus extra for steaks

½ bunch fresh thyme sprigs

4 x beef rib-eye steaks

Mustard, to serve

Method

1. Preheat oven to 200°C/180°C. Line two oven trays with baking paper. Combine sweet potatoes evenly on trays. Toss with olive oil to coat and season. Bake for 35-40 minutes until golden and tender

2. Meanwhile, drizzle steaks with extra oil. Sprinkle both sides with salt and pepper. Cook steaks in a large oven-proof frying pan over medium-high heat for 2-3 minutes each side until browned. Transfer pan to oven and cook for about 5 minutes until cooked to taste. Rest steaks for 5 minutes

3. Serve steaks with potato medley and mustard

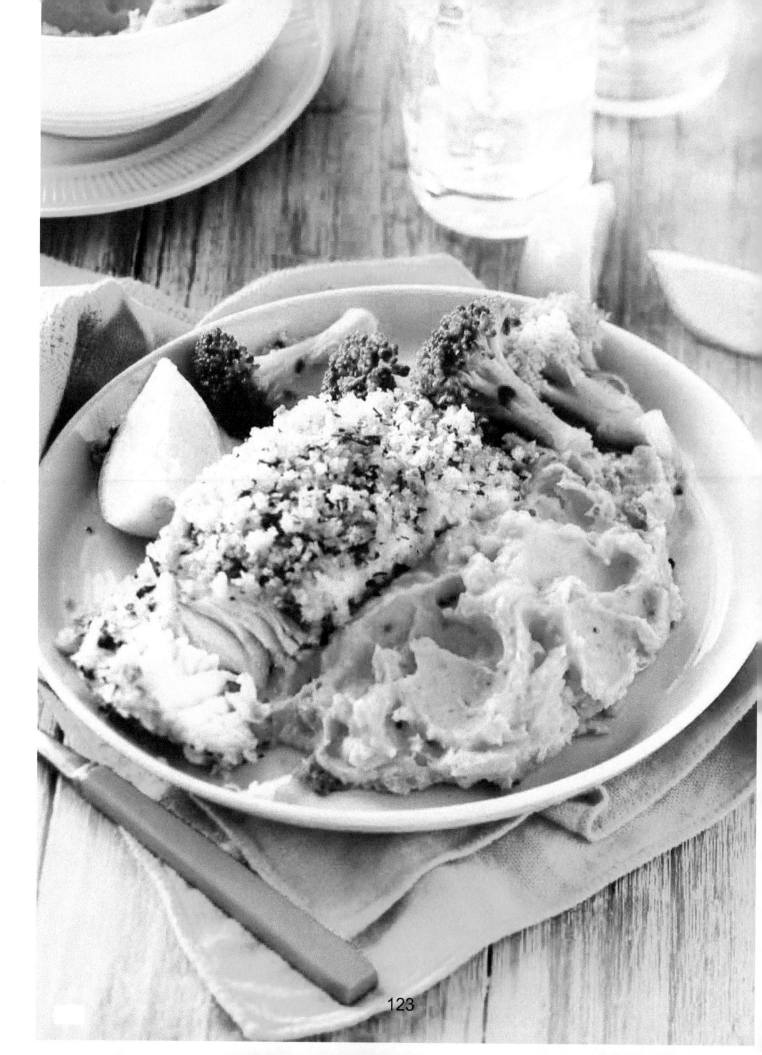

LEMON AND HERB FISH WITH SWEET POTATO MASH

Prep Time: 20 minutes
Cook Time: 1 hour
Serves: 4

Ingredients

600g Sweet Potato, peeled, chopped

¼ cup (60g) light sour cream

3 teaspoons wholegrain mustard

3/4 cup sourdough breadcrumbs

1/3 cup (40g) grated parmesan

1 tablespoon chopped parsley

1 teaspoon finely grated lemon rind

3 teaspoons olive oil

4 x 120g barramundi fillets, skin off

250g steamed broccoli florets, to serve

Method

1. Preheat oven to 200°C/180°C fan-forced

2. Boil, steam or microwave sweet potato until tender. Mash with sour cream and mustard. Season to taste

3. Meanwhile, combine breadcrumbs, parmesan, parsley, lemon and oil in a bowl. Mix well

4. Place fish on a baking paper-lined tray. Coat fish with crumb mixture. Bake for 15-20 minutes until fish flakes easily with a fork

5. Serve fish with mash and broccoli

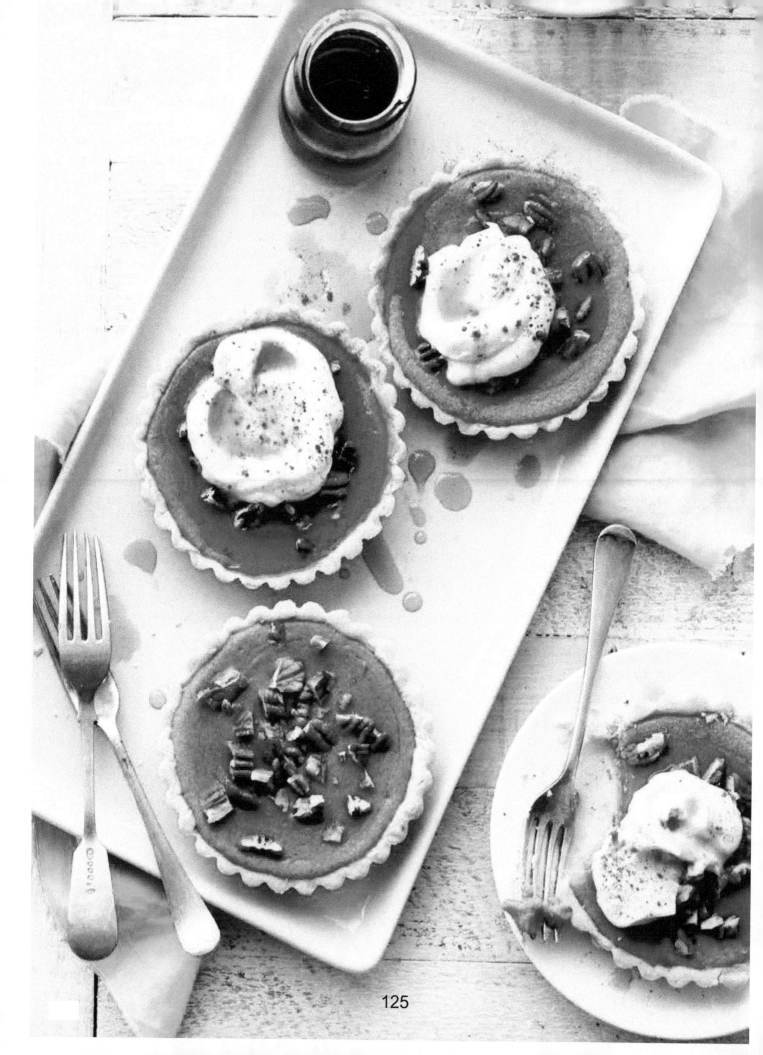

SWEET POTATO AND PECAN PIES

Prep Time: 35 minutes
Cook Time: 45 minutes
Makes: 6

Ingredients

PASTRY

1½ cups (225g) plain flour

2 tablespoons icing sugar

125g cold butter, chopped

1 egg yolk

1-2 tablespoons iced water

FILLING

500g Sweet Potato, peeled, chopped

½ cup (110g) brown sugar

1 teaspoon vanilla bean paste

1 teaspoon cinnamon

½ teaspoon ground ginger

¼ teaspoon nutmeg

1 cup (250ml) pouring cream

2 eggs

½ cup chopped pecans

Whipped cream and maple syrup, to serve

Method

PASTRY

1. Grease six 10cm loose based fluted tart tins

2. Process flour, icing sugar and butter until crumbly. Add egg yolk and enough of the water to make dough come together. Knead dough on floured surface until smooth. Wrap in plastic and chill for 30 minutes

3. Preheat oven to 200°C /180°C. Meanwhile, steam sweet potato until tender. Cool 10 minutes

4. Divide pastry into six portions. Roll out each and line tins. Chill for 15 minutes. Line pastry with baking paper, fill with dried beans or rice. Bake 10 minutes; remove paper and beans. Bake 5 minutes or until browned lightly

5. Reduce oven to 180°C /160°C

FILLING

1. Blend or process sweet potato with sugar, paste, spices, cream and eggs until smooth. Pour mixture into pastry cases. Sprinkle with pecans

2. Bake for 25-30 minutes until set. Cool to room temperature before chilling until firm. Serve topped with whipped cream and a drizzle of maple syrup

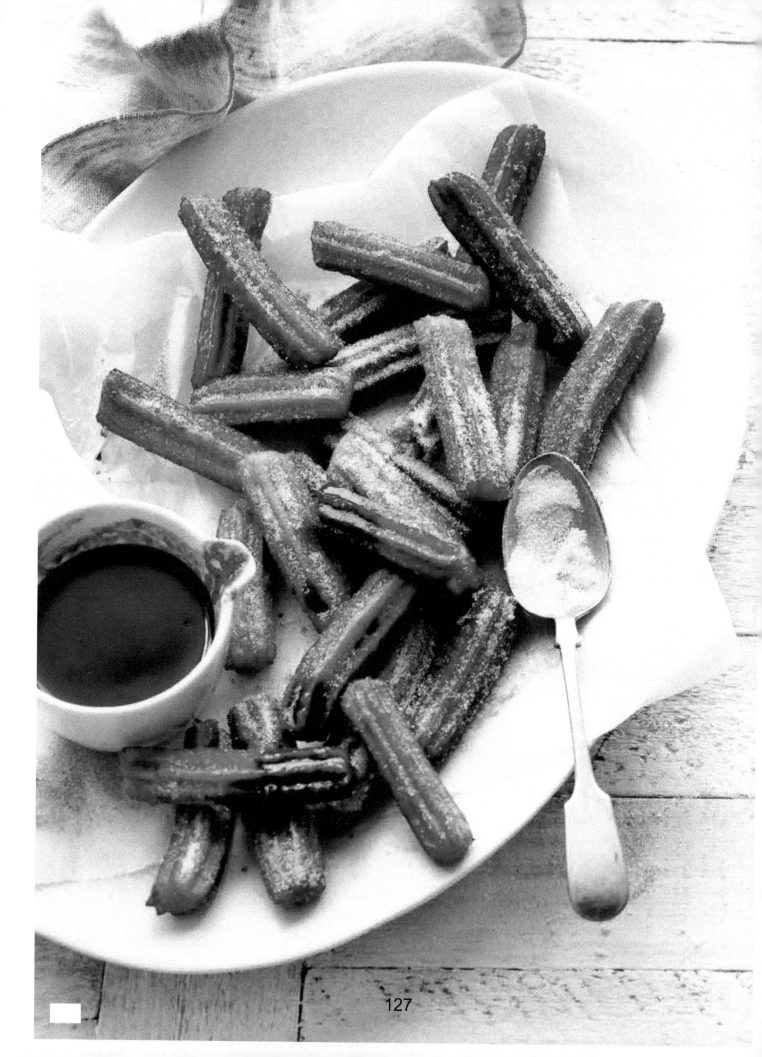

SWEET POTATO CHURROS WITH CACAO DIPPING SAUCE

Prep Time: 25 minutes
Cook Time: 20 minutes
Makes: Approximately 35

Ingredients

SWEET POTATO CHURROS

¾ cup (185ml) water

60g butter

¾ cup (110g) plain flour

Pinch salt

½ teaspoon cinnamon, plus 1 teaspoon, extra for dusting

Pinch nutmeg

½ cup Sweet Potato puree

2 eggs

Vegetable oil, for deep-frying

¼ cup (55g) caster sugar

RAW CHOCOLATE SAUCE

3 tablespoons rice malt syrup

2 tablespoons coconut oil

1½ tablespoons cacao powder

1 teaspoon vanilla extract

Method

SWEET POTATO CHURROS

1. Preheat oven to 200°C /180°C fan-forced

2. Combine water and butter in a medium saucepan and bring to the boil over high heat until butter melts. Add flour, salt and spices and stir with a wooden spoon until dough comes away from the side of pan

3. Remove from heat. Add puree, stirring until combined. Cool 5 minutes

4. Add eggs, one at a time, beating well after each addition until well combined. Spoon dough into a piping bag fitted with a 1.5cm star nozzle

5. Add enough oil in a large saucepan until 6cm deep. Heat oil to 180°C over medium heat. Pipe 7cm lengths of dough into the oil cutting dough with a small sharp knife or scissors. Deep-fry for 2-3 minutes until golden brown

6. Using a slotted spoon, transfer churros to a plate lined with paper towel. Dust with combined sugar and extra cinnamon. Repeat with remaining dough, in batches

RAW CHOCOLATE SAUCE

1. Melt coconut oil in small pan. Stir in syrup, cacao and vanilla until smooth. Serve churros with sauce

Tips

Chill chocolate sauce, if you prefer a thicker sauce.

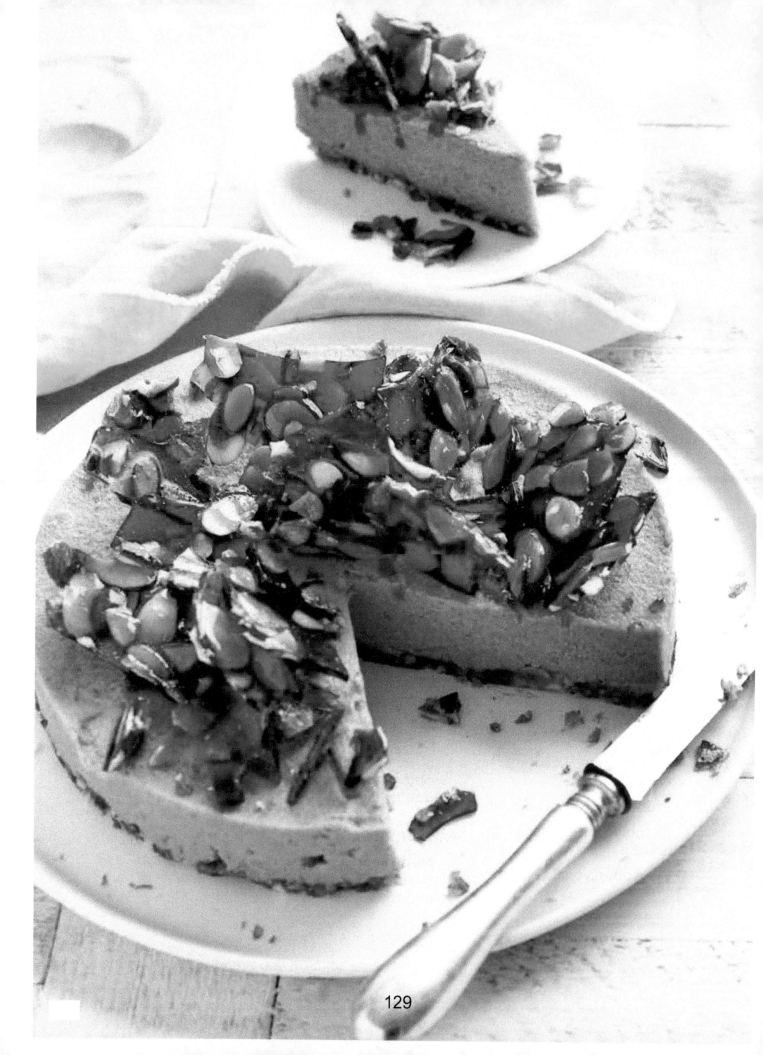

SWEET POTATO VEGAN CHEESECAKE

Prep Time: 30 minutes, plus soaking time and freezing time

Cook Time: 1 hour 15 minutes

Serves: 12

Ingredients

CHEESECAKE

500g Sweet Potato

½ cup (80g) whole almonds (with skin)

100g medjool dates, pitted (for base)

2 cups cashews, soaked overnight

¼ cup (60ml) coconut oil

80g medjool dates, pitted (for filling)

½ cup (125ml) rice malt syrup

2 tablespoons lemon juice

2 teaspoons vanilla bean paste

1½ tsp ground cinnamon

½ tsp mixed spice

¼ teaspoon ground ginger

PRALINE

½ cup natural sliced almonds, toasted

1 cup caster sugar

⅓ cup water

Method

CHEESECAKE

1. Preheat oven to 200°C /180°C fan-forced. Prick sweet potato all over with a small knife. Spray with oil and place on a tray. Bake for about an hour or until tender. Cool slightly before removing skin

2. Combine almonds and dates in a food processor. Process until fine and sticky. Using damp hands, press mixture into a lined 20cm spring form pan. Chill until needed

3. Drain cashews and place in a food processor with oil, dates, syrup, juice, paste and spices. Process until completely smooth (this may take a few minutes). Add sweet potato and process until combined. Pour over almond base in pan

4. Level top and freeze, covered for 4 hours or overnight until firm. Once firm, transfer to fridge

PRALINE

1. Scatter almonds over a baking paper-lined tray. Combine sugar and water in a saucepan over low heat. Cook, stirring, for 5 minutes or until sugar has dissolved. Increase heat to high. Bring to the boil. Boil, without stirring, for about 5-8 minutes until mixture turns golden

2. Remove from heat and let bubbles subside. Pour over almonds. Allow to cool. Break into shards

3. Serve cheesecake topped with praline shards

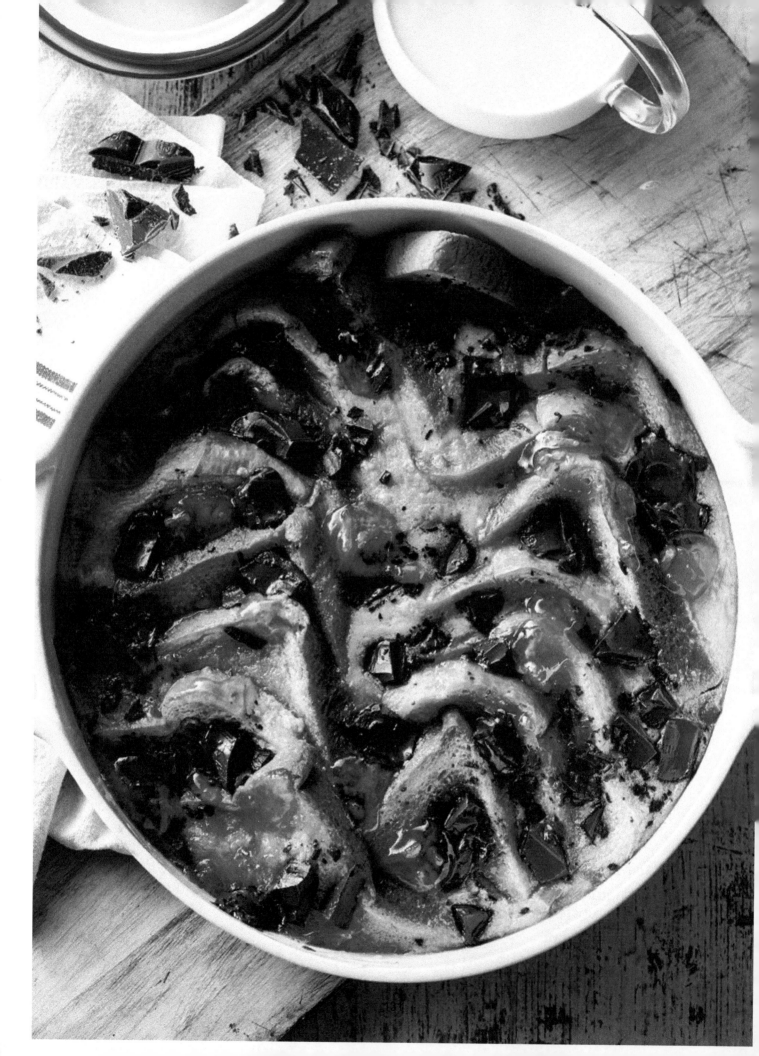

CHOC-ORANGE 'BREAD & BUTTER' *pudding*

 PREP 15 MINS   **COOK** 50-60 MINS **SERVES** 6-8

INGREDIENTS

8 slices brioche loaf

80 g (about ⅓ cup) Western Star Spreadable Original Soft

½ cup orange or blood orange marmalade

600 ml Western Star Thickened Cream, plus extra, to serve

4 eggs

½ cup brown sugar

2 teaspoons vanilla

100g dark or milk chocolate, chopped into chunks

METHOD

1. Preheat oven to 160°C / 145°C fan-forced.

2. Spread both sides of the brioche slices with the Spreadable, then spread only one side of each slice with the marmalade. Cut each slice in half and place overlapping, marmalade side up, into the base of a round 8-cup capacity baking dish.

3. In a bowl, whisk together the cream, eggs, brown sugar and vanilla then pour over the bread. Dot the chocolate chunks among the brioche slices, then stand for 10 minutes.

4. Bake for 50-60 minutes or until the custard has just set. Serve warm with extra cream.

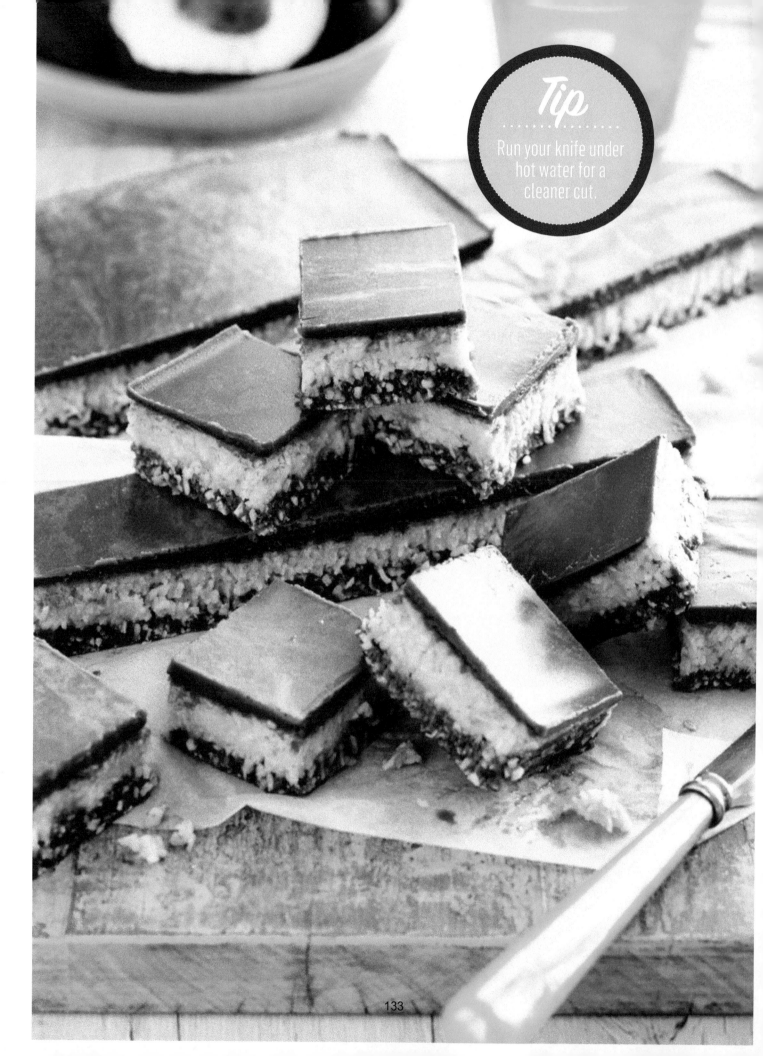

Tip

Run your knife under hot water for a cleaner cut.

RAW AVOCADO
slice

 PREP 15 MINS + FREEZER TIME 👤 **MAKES** 24

INGREDIENTS

BASE

1 cup raw cashews

1 cup oats (LOWAN)

1 packet fresh pitted medjool dates

2 tbs cacao powder

¼ coconut oil, melted

AVOCADO FILLING

4 cups shredded coconut

1 tbs coconut sugar

¼ cup Natvia

2 Avocados

¾ cup coconut oil, melted
and cooled

CHOC TOP

2 tablespoons cacao powder

⅔ cup coconut oil, melted
and cooled

⅓ cup maple syrup

METHOD

BASE

1. Put cashews and oats in a food processor and blitz to make a rough crumb (not too chunky). Add the dates, cacao and a pinch of salt. Blend the mixture and slowly add the coconut oil to bring the mix together. You may not need all the coconut oil. Press mix evenly into a slice pan, lined with baking paper and transfer to the freezer to firm up.

AVOCADO FILLING

1. Place all ingredients in a clean food processor bowl and blitz to combine to desired consistency. Add to prepared base. Return to freezer to set for at least 30 minutes before adding the chocolate top.

CHOC TOP

1. Combine all ingredients in a bowl and pour over the top of avocado slice. Return slice to freezer for 1-2 hours until slice is completely set.

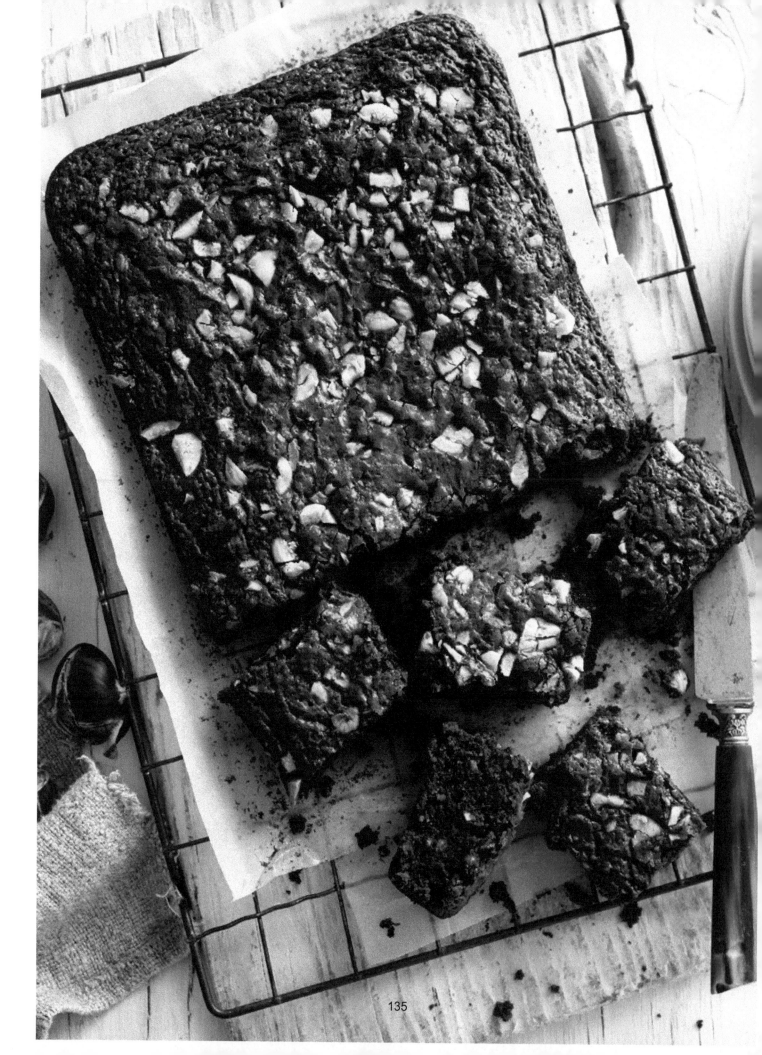

GLUTEN-FREE CHESTNUT
& chocolate brownies

 PREP 20 MINS   **COOK** 25-30 MINS   **MAKES** 16

INGREDIENTS

CHESTNUTS

500g fresh chestnuts

BROWNIES

350g cooked and peeled chestnuts

Standard self-raising flour can be used for a non-gluten free version.

200g good quality dark chocolate, broken into squares

200g unsalted butter, chopped

1 ¼ cups brown sugar

1 tsp vanilla extract

4 eggs, lightly beaten

½ cup gluten-free self-raising flour

2 tbsp cocoa

Pinch salt

METHOD

CHESTNUTS

1. Preheat oven to 200°C / 180°C fan-forced.

2. Cut a shallow cross into the flat side of each chestnut shell. Place prepared chestnuts onto a baking tray and bake for 15 to 20 minutes or until the shells split open.

3. Remove chestnuts from the heat and wrap in a clean tea towel for 5 minutes. While chestnuts are still warm, quickly peel off the outer brown shell and remove the papery thin skin underneath.

BROWNIES

1. Reduce oven to 180°C / 160°C fan-forced. Grease and line a 16cm x 26cm x 2-3cm deep slab pan with baking paper, leaving a 2cm overhang on the sides.

2. Set aside 50g cooked and peeled chestnuts. Place remaining chestnuts into a food processor. Process until fine crumbs form (you'll need 2 cups ground chestnuts). Set aside.

3. Place chocolate and butter in a large microwave safe bowl and microwave on high for 2 minutes, stirring with a metal spoon every minute until melted. Set aside to cool.

4. Using a metal spoon, stir in sugar, vanilla and eggs into chocolate mixture until well combined. Sift over flour, cocoa and salt. Stir to combine. Gently fold through chestnuts. Pour into prepared pan. Chop reserved chestnuts and sprinkle over mixture. Bake for 25-30 minutes until a skewer inserted comes out with moist crumbs sticking. Cool completely in the pan. Cut into squares. Serve with whipped cream and a dusting of cocoa if liked.

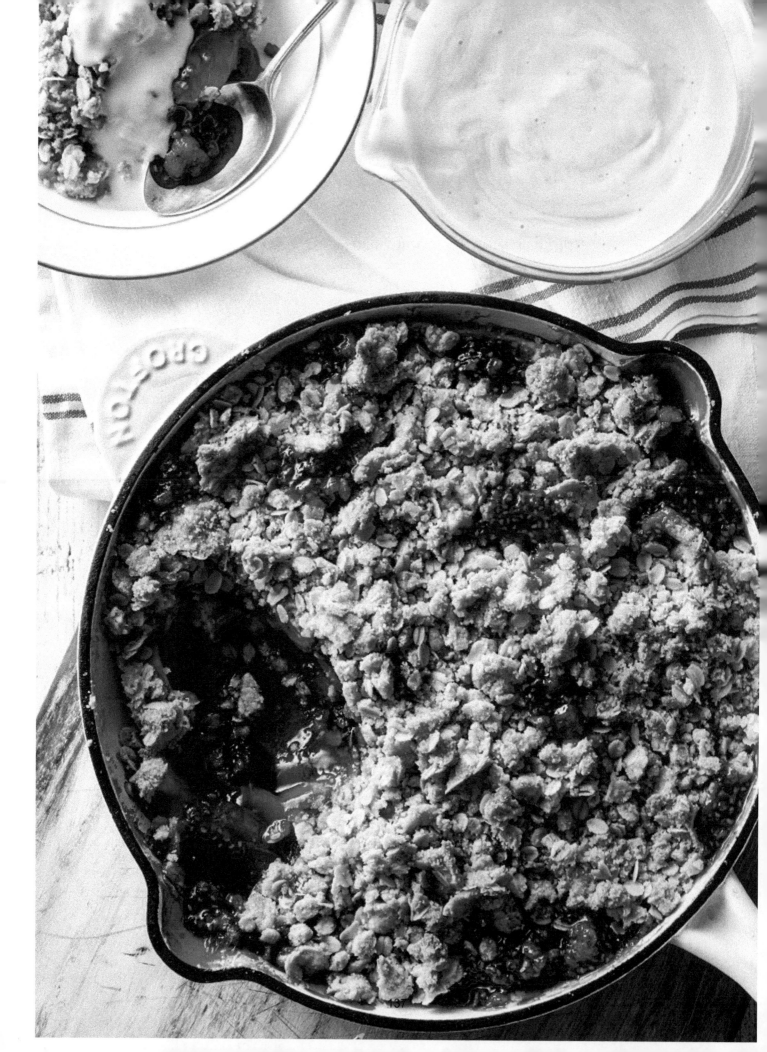

APPLE & MIXED BERRY CRUMBLE
with orange custard

 PREP 20 MINS **COOK** 45 MINS 👤 **SERVES** 6

INGREDIENTS

APPLE-BERRY MIXTURE

60 g Western Star Chef's Choice Unsalted Cultured Butter

¼ cup caster sugar

4 granny smith apples, peeled, quartered and sliced into 3

3 cups frozen mixed berries, thawed and drained

CRUMBLE TOPPING

1 ½ cups plain flour

1 cup oats

¾ cup light brown sugar

¼ teaspoon ground cinnamon

¼ teaspoon salt

150 g Western Star Chef's Choice Cultured Unsalted Butter, cut into cubes

ORANGE CUSTARD

300 ml bottle Western Star Thickened Cream

1 orange, rind zested

2 egg yolks

¼ cup caster sugar

2 teaspoons cornflour

METHOD

APPLE-BERRY MIXTURE

1. In a medium (about 2 litre capacity) oven-proof frying pan, combine the butter and sugar. Cook over medium heat, stirring, until melted and combined. Add the apple and toss well to coat. Cover with the lid and simmer for 10 minutes, stirring occasionally. Toss through the mixed berries.

CRUMBLE TOPPING

2. Preheat oven to 200°C / 185°C fan-forced. Place the flour, oats, sugar, cinnamon and salt in a large bowl, and use your fingertips to rub the Butter into the dry ingredients until large clumps form. Scatter over the berry mixture to evenly coat.

3. Bake in oven for 30-35 minutes or until top is golden and juice is bubbling.

4. While the crumble is cooking, make the orange custard.

ORANGE CUSTARD

5. Pour the cream into a small saucepan over medium-low heat. Add almost all the orange zest (reserving a small amount to garnish) and stir to combine. Bring to just before boiling point and turn off heat.

6. Place the egg yolks, sugar and cornflour in a large heat-proof bowl. Use a balloon whisk to whisk until pale and creamy. Gradually pour the hot cream mixture into the egg yolk mixture, whisking constantly, until combined and smooth. Return to the saucepan over very low heat. Stir constantly for about 5 minutes or until custard is thickened and coats the back of a wooden spoon.

7. Serve the crumble with the orange custard and sprinkled with reserved orange zest.

Top Tip

Press Hass avocados near the stem to check if they're ripe. They should give a little.

DAIRY-FREE LEMON AVOCADO
pound cake

 PREP 15 MINS **COOK** 50 MINS 👤 **SERVES** 8

INGREDIENTS

AVOCADO CAKE

1¼ cups plain wholemeal flour

¼ cup cornflour

1 tablespoon baking powder

1 cup raw caster sugar

½ cup desiccated coconut

¼ cup coconut oil

2 eggs

2 teaspoons finely grated lemon rind

2 medium avocados, mashed
(1¼ cups mashed)

½ cup coconut milk

¼ cup shredded coconut

COCONUT ICING

400ml tin coconut cream

1½ tablespoons honey

METHOD

AVOCADO CAKE

1. Preheat oven to 180°C / 160°C fan-forced and line a loaf tin with baking paper.

2. Place the flour, cornflour, baking powder, sugar and coconut in a large bowl and mix together. Make a well in the centre and add the oil, eggs, lemon rind, avocado and coconut milk. Whisk until just combined.

3. Pour into loaf tin and bake for 50 minutes, or until a skewer inserted into the centre comes out clean. Allow to cool in tin completely.

4. Meanwhile, make the icing.

5. When ready to serve, spoon the icing over the cake and scatter with shredded coconut.

COCONUT ICING

6. Place the coconut cream in the fridge for 24 hours. Once chilled completely, remove the top firm creamy layer and place in a large bowl (you should have about ¾ cup).

TIPS & HINTS:

Coconut cream varies in consistency from brand to brand and after refrigeration, some coconut creams may be thicker than others. If your icing is very thick, add a few tablespoons of coconut milk or water to thin the icing.

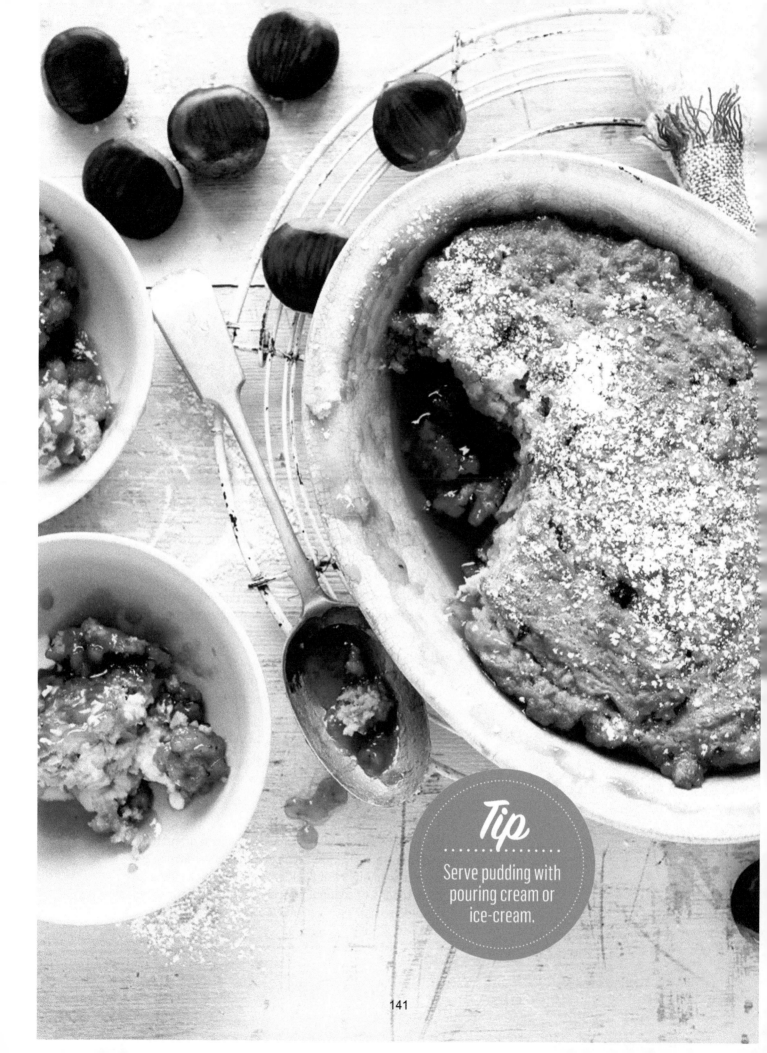

Tip

Serve pudding with pouring cream or ice-cream.

CHESTNUT & GOLDEN SYRUP
pudding

 PREP 20 MINS   **COOK** 50 MINS   **SERVES** 4-6

INGREDIENTS

220g fresh chestnuts

½ cup milk

1 egg

80g butter, melted

2 tbsp golden syrup

⅓ cup firmly-packed brown sugar

1¼ cups self-raising flour, sifted

½ cup brown sugar

2 tsp cornflour

1¼ cups boiling water

¼ cup golden syrup

Icing sugar, for dusting

METHOD

1. Cut chestnuts in half across the width of the chestnut.

2. Place prepared chestnuts into a saucepan of cold water and bring to the boil.

3. Simmer for 15-20 minutes. Remove the chestnuts one at a time from the water.

4. Wrap in a clean tea towel for 5-10 minutes. While chestnuts are still warm, quickly peel off the outer brown shell and remove the papery thin skin underneath.

5. Preheat oven to 180°C / 160°C fan-forced. Lightly grease an 8-cup deep ovenproof dish.

6. Finely grate chestnuts in a food processor. In a large bowl, combine milk, egg, butter and golden syrup. Stir in chestnuts, sugar and sifted flour. Using a large metal spoon, mix until just combined. Spoon into the prepared dish.

7. To make the sauce, combine sugar and cornflour in a small bowl. Sprinkle over pudding. Combine water and golden syrup in a jug. Pour mixture over the back of large metal spoon over the pudding batter. Place dish on a baking tray lined with baking paper.

8. Bake for 50-55 minutes until golden and pudding bounces back when gently pressed in the centre. Stand for 5 minutes. Dust with icing sugar.

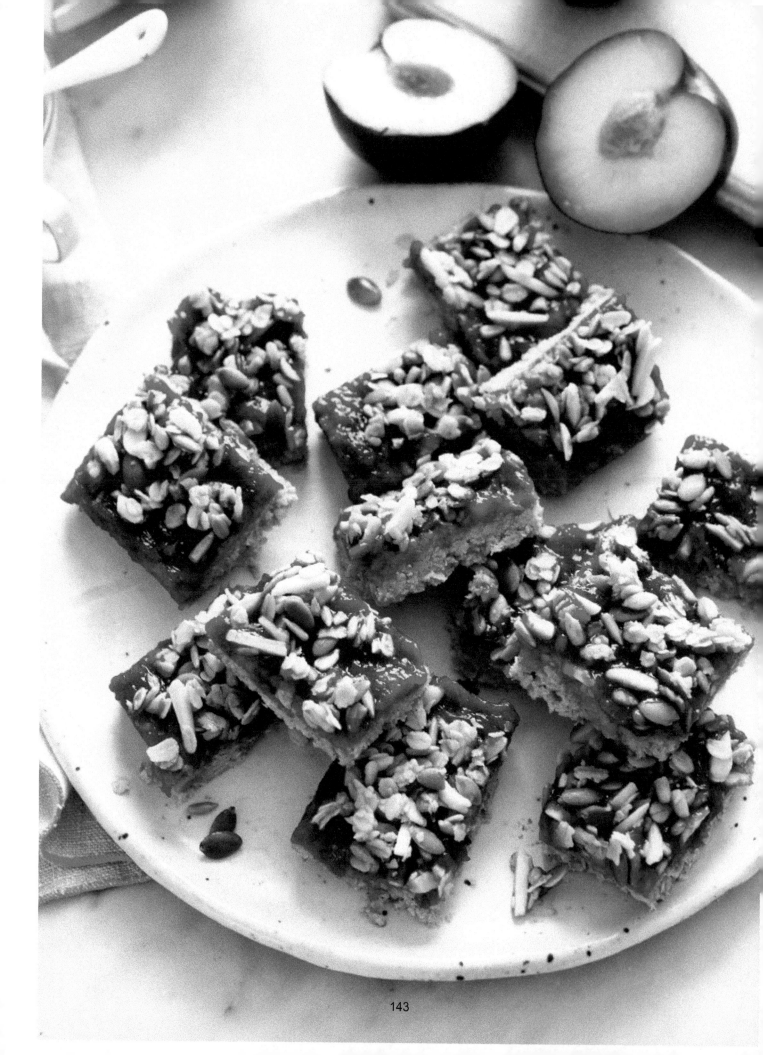

HEALTHY PLUM
slice

 PREP 20 MINS   **COOK** 55 MINS **MAKES** 12

INGREDIENTS

Filling

6 plums, stones removed, roughly chopped

2 tablespoons maple syrup

Base

2 cups rolled oats

1 cup almond meal

¼ cup maple syrup

2 tablespoons coconut oil

1 teaspoon sea salt flakes

1 teaspoon cinnamon

Topping

½ cup rolled oats

¼ cup slivered almonds

¼ cup pumpkin seeds

2 tablespoons sunflower seeds

1 tablespoon coconut oil

METHOD

Filling

1. Place plums and maple syrup into a saucepan and place over a medium heat. Bring mixture to the boil and simmer for 15-20 minutes until plums are soft, pulpy and firm. Cool. Place in fridge until required. (This can be made the day or night ahead of making.)

Base

1. Preheat oven to 180°C. Grease and line a 20cm x 20cm cake pan with baking paper.

2. To make the base place oats, almond meal, maple syrup, coconut oil, salt and cinnamon into a food processor and process until well combined and finely chopped. Press evenly over base of prepared cake pan. Bake for 15 minutes. Cool.

Topping

1. Spread plum mixture over cold base. For topping, combine oats, almonds, pumpkin seeds, sunflower seeds and coconut oil in a bowl. Stir until combined.

2. Sprinkle mixture over plums, pressing lightly. Bake for 20 minutes or until topping is light golden. Cool in pan. Remove from pan and cut into bars or squares.

3. Store in an airtight container in the refrigerator for up to 5 days.

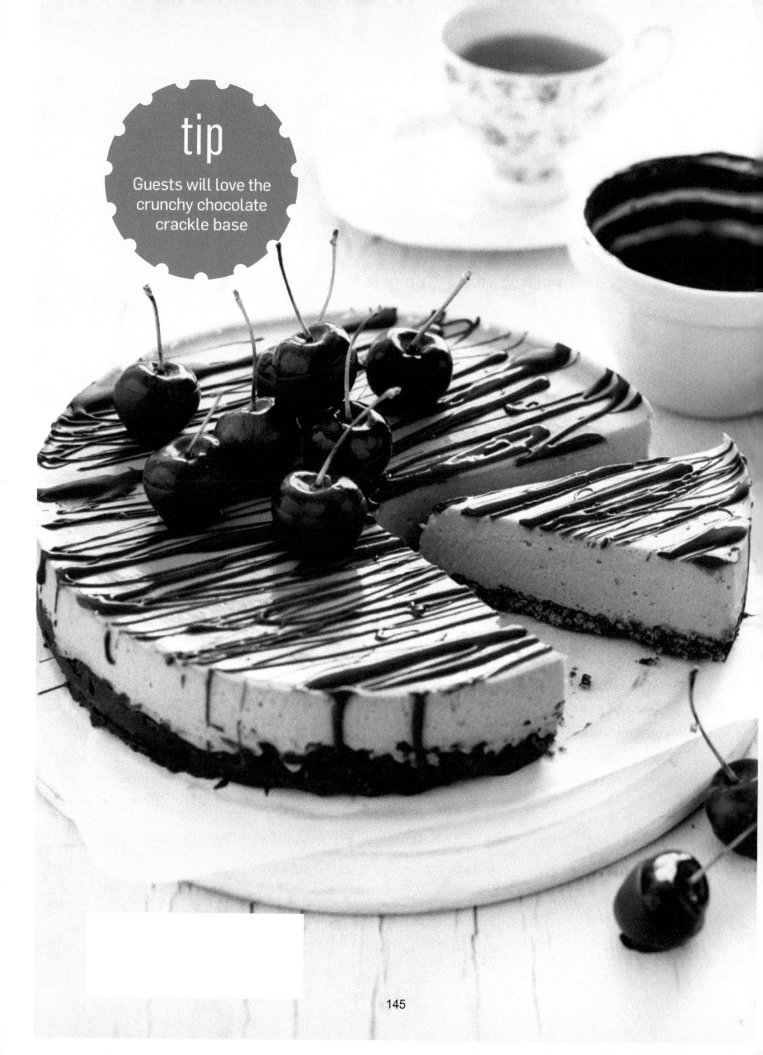

CHERRY COCONUT CHEESECAKE WITH
chocolate crackle base

PREP 30 MINS, PLUS 1 HOUR, 15 MINS SETTING TIME **SERVES** 12

INGREDIENTS

CHOCOLATE CRACKLE BASE

60g (¼ cup) Copha, chopped

60g dark chocolate, chopped

80g (½ cup) icing sugar mixture, sifted

2 tablespoons cocoa powder

50g (1 ⅔ cup) Kellogg's Rice Bubbles

20g (⅓ cup) desiccated coconut

CHEESECAKE FILLING

300g (1 ½ cups) cherries, pitted and halved

60ml (¼ cup) water

160g (1 cup) icing sugar mixture, sifted

500g cream cheese, chopped and softened

270ml can coconut cream

3 teaspoons powdered gelatine

CHOC-CHERRY TOPPING

100g dark chocolate, chopped

20g (1 tablespoon) Copha

12 cherries, extra

METHOD

CHOCOLATE CRACKLE BASE

1. Grease and line the base and sides of a 22cm spring form cake tin. In a heatproof bowl, combine chocolate and Copha. Place over a pot of lightly simmering water. Stir until melted. Remove from heat.

2. Place sugar, cocoa, rice bubbles and coconut in a large bowl. Add Copha mixture and mix to combine. Press into base of tin. Put in fridge to set for 10 minutes.

CHEESECAKE FILLING

3. Place cherries, sugar, water in a small saucepan over high heat. Bring to the boil and cook for 4 minutes, to soften. Remove from the heat and cool slightly for 5 minutes. Using a stick blender, blend until smooth.

4. Sprinkle over the gelatine and set aside for 5 minutes to dissolve. Mix until smooth. Set aside.

5. Place cheese in large bowl and using hand-held beaters, beat for 4 minutes until light and fluffy. Add coconut cream and beat for 4 minutes until light and smooth. Strain the cherry mixture through a sieve and gradually add to the cheese mixture. Stir to combine. Pour over base and put in fridge to set for 1 hour.

CHOC-CHERRY TOPPING

6. In a heatproof bowl, combine the chocolate and Copha. Place over a pot of lightly simmering water. Stir occasionally until melted. Remove from heat.

7. Half dip the cherries in the chocolate, place on baking paper and refrigerate for 2 minutes to set.

1. Remove cheesecake from tin and drizzle with chocolate mixture. Top with cherries to serve.

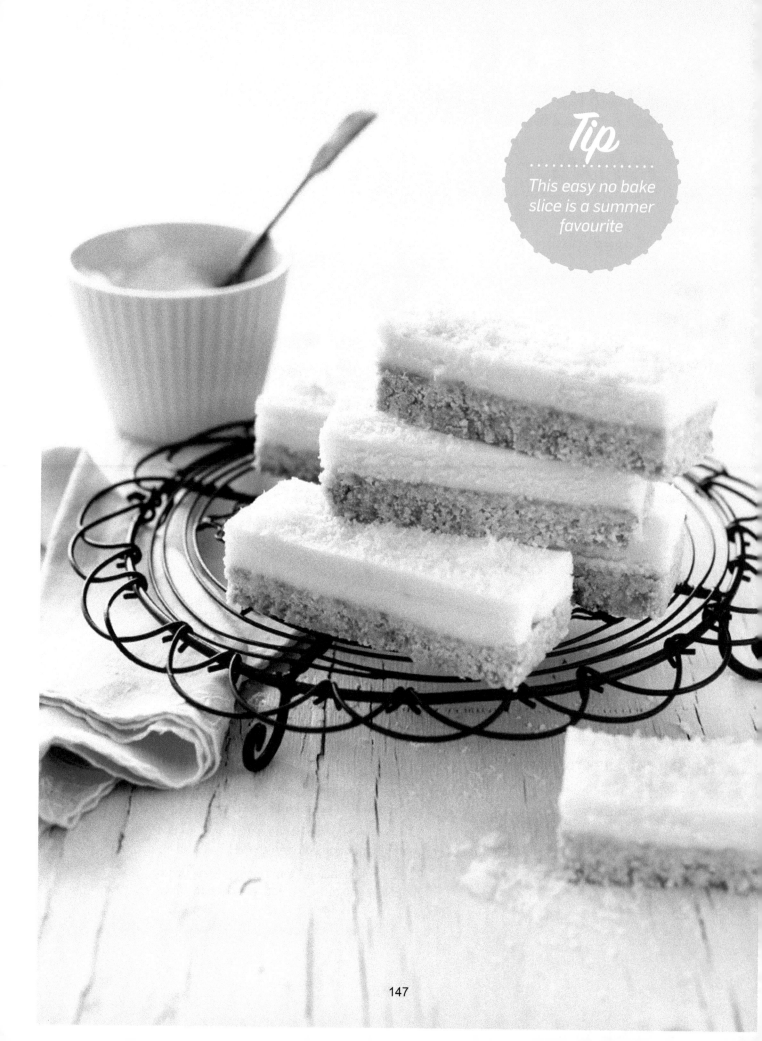

Tip

This easy no bake slice is a summer favourite

147

LEMON COCONUT
slice

 PREP 30 MINS   👤 **MAKES** 24 BARS

INGREDIENTS

BASE

125g (½ block) Copha, chopped

250g (1 packet) Arnott's Milk Coffee Biscuits

80g (1 cup) desiccated coconut

160g (½ cup) sweetened condensed milk

LEMON TOPPING

185g (¾ cup) Copha, chopped

110g (¾ cup) white chocolate melts

200g (⅔ cup) sweetened condensed milk

250g tub sour cream

60ml (¼ cup) lemon juice

2 teaspoons finely grated lemon rind

40g (½ cup) desiccated coconut, extra

1 teaspoon finely grated lemon rind, extra

METHOD

BASE

1. Grease and line a 20cm x 30cm slice tin. Make sure the paper has a 2cm overhang

2. Melt the Copha in a microwave on high or in a saucepan until fully melted. Using a food processor process the biscuits and coconut until they resemble fine breadcrumbs

3. Add the melted Copha and sweetened condensed milk and mix together. Press the biscuit mixture firmly into the tin, using the back of a spoon. Put in the fridge to set for 10 minutes

LEMON TOPPING

1. Melt the Copha and chocolate in a microwave on high or in a saucepan over low heat until fully melted and combined

2. Place sweetened condensed milk, sour cream, lemon juice and rind in a large bowl and mix to combine. Add the Copha chocolate mixture and mix until smooth

3. Pour over the base and smooth the top. Put in the fridge to set for 20 minutes

4. Place extra coconut and lemon rind in a small bowl and mix to combine. Sprinkle over the slice to serve. Slice into 24 bars

TIPS & HINTS

This slice will keep in an airtight container in the fridge for up to 3 days

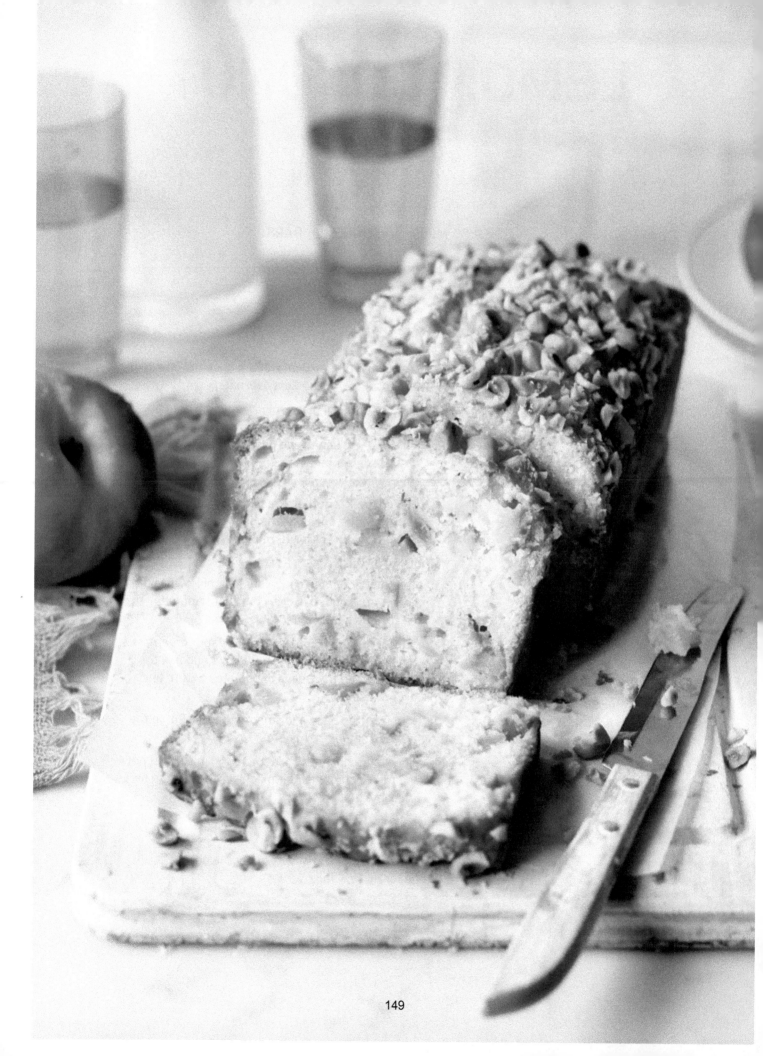

PEACH, COCONUT AND HAZELNUT *loaf*

 PREP 15 MINS **COOK** 10 MINS 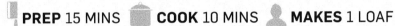 **MAKES** 1 LOAF

INGREDIENTS

125g butter, softened

⅔ cup caster sugar

1 teaspoon vanilla extract

2 eggs, at room temperature

1 cup sour cream

2 yellow peaches, stone removed, finely diced

1½ cups self-raising flour

½ cup plain flour

½ cup desiccated coconut

⅓ cup roasted hazelnuts, finely chopped

METHOD

1. Preheat oven to 180°C. Grease a 6 cup-capacity (20cm x 10cm x 7cm deep base measurement) loaf pan and line with baking paper, 5cm above line of pan. Using an electric mixer, beat butter, sugar and vanilla until pale and creamy. Add egg, 1 at a time, beating well after each addition.

2. Using a large metal spoon, gently fold in sour cream, peaches and coconut. Sift flours over batter and gently fold until combined.

3. Spoon batter into prepared loaf pan. Smooth top and sprinkle with chopped nuts, pressing gently into batter. Bake for 1 hour or until a skewer inserted into the centre comes out clean. Stand for 10 minutes before turning out onto a wire rack to cool.

Tip

You can swap
out the nectarines
for peaches

151

NECTARINE AND APRICOT COCONUT
chia puddings

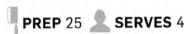 **PREP** 25 **SERVES** 4

INGREDIENTS

2 x 270m cans coconut milk

¾ cup white chia seeds

1 teaspoon vanilla extract

4 yellow nectarines, stone removed, cut into thin wedges

4 apricots, stone removed, finely diced

½ cup maple syrup, to serve

¼ cup toasted flaked coconut, to serve

METHOD

1. Place coconut milk, chia seeds and vanilla into a bowl and stir until well combined. Set aside for 15 minutes to thicken.

2. Spoon half the chia mixture into the base of 4 x 1 cup-capacity glasses or glass bowls. Top with half the nectarines and apricots. Spoon remaining chia seed mixture over fruit. Place remaining fruit onto chia seed mixture.

3. Place in refrigerator for 1 hour or until cold. Drizzle the maple syrup over the fruit. Sprinkle with coconut and serve.

NO-BAKE BLUEBERRY & SWEET RICOTTA *tart*

 PREP 25 MINS + CHILLING TIME **SERVES** 8

INGREDIENTS

Biscuit base

250g Butternut Snap or Marie biscuits

125g unsalted butter, melted

Ricotta cannoli filling

500g fresh ricotta

⅓ cup icing sugar, plus extra for dusting

½ tsp vanilla extract

250g blueberries

Finely shredded orange zest and honey, to serve

METHOD

1. To make the biscuit base, place biscuits into a food processor and process until finely chopped. Add butter and process until well combined.

2. Evenly press mixture into the base of 22cm wide x 2.5cm deep loose-base fluted tart pan. Refrigerate for 3 hours (or longer if time permits).

3. To make the filling, place ricotta, icing sugar and vanilla into a medium bowl. Using electric hand beaters, beat the mixture until smooth. Cover and chill until ready to serve.

4. Just before serving, fill the tart case with the ricotta mixture. Scatter with blueberries. Dust with icing sugar and sprinkle with orange zest. Drizzle with a little honey and serve.

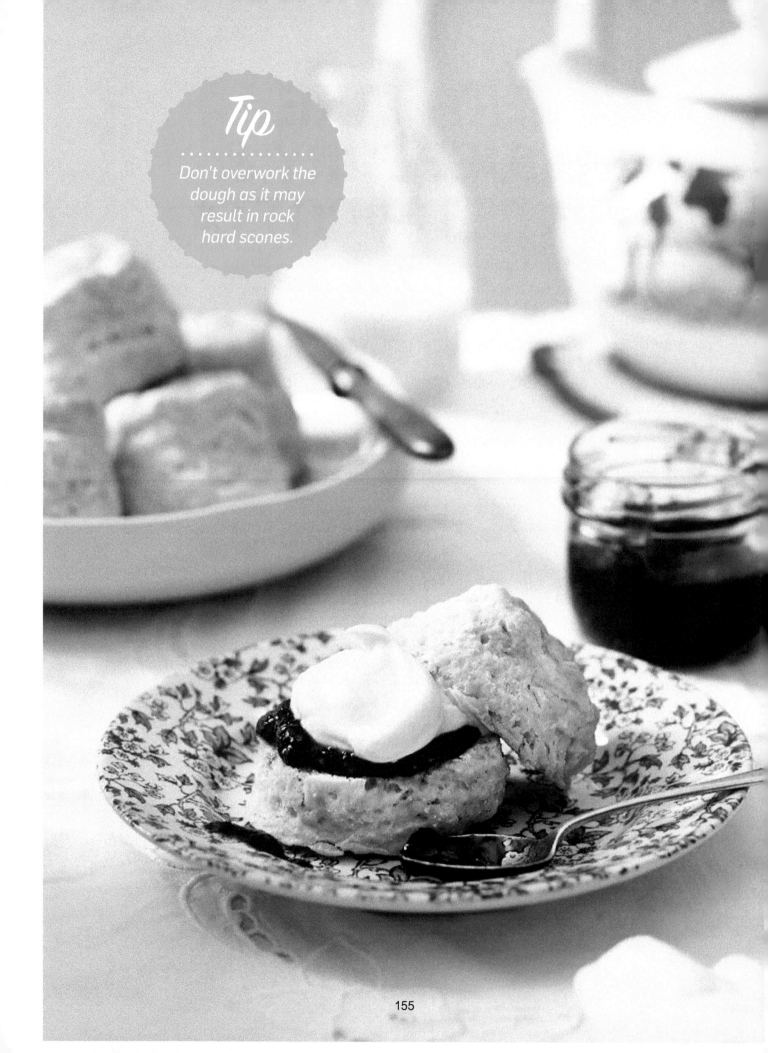

LEMONADE
scones

 PREP 10-12 MINS   **COOK** 15 MINS **MAKES** 12 SLICES

INGREDIENTS

LEMONADE SCONES

3 cups self-raising flour

½ tsp baking powder

1 tsp sugar

60g Copha

300ml lemonade

Plain flour, for kneading
and rolling

1 egg, beaten

METHOD

1. Pre-heat oven to 190°C
2. In a large bowl, combine the self-raising flour, baking powder and sugar
3. Grate the Copha over the flour. Rub the Copha into the flour until mixture resembles fine breadcrumbs
4. Make a well in the centre of the flour mixture and pour in ¾ of the lemonade. Mix to a firm but tacky dough, adding more lemonade if required
5. Turn dough out onto a lightly floured board and knead gently
6. Roll dough out to a 4cm thick circle
7. Using a floured cutter, cut out scones. Re-roll dough as required
8. Place scones onto a floured non-stick baking tray. Brush scones with beaten egg and bake in the pre-heated oven at 190°C for 12-15 minutes
9. Cool on a wire rack and serve warm

TIPS & HINTS:

If making date or sultana scones, add ½ cup of fruit and 1 beaten egg to the mixture

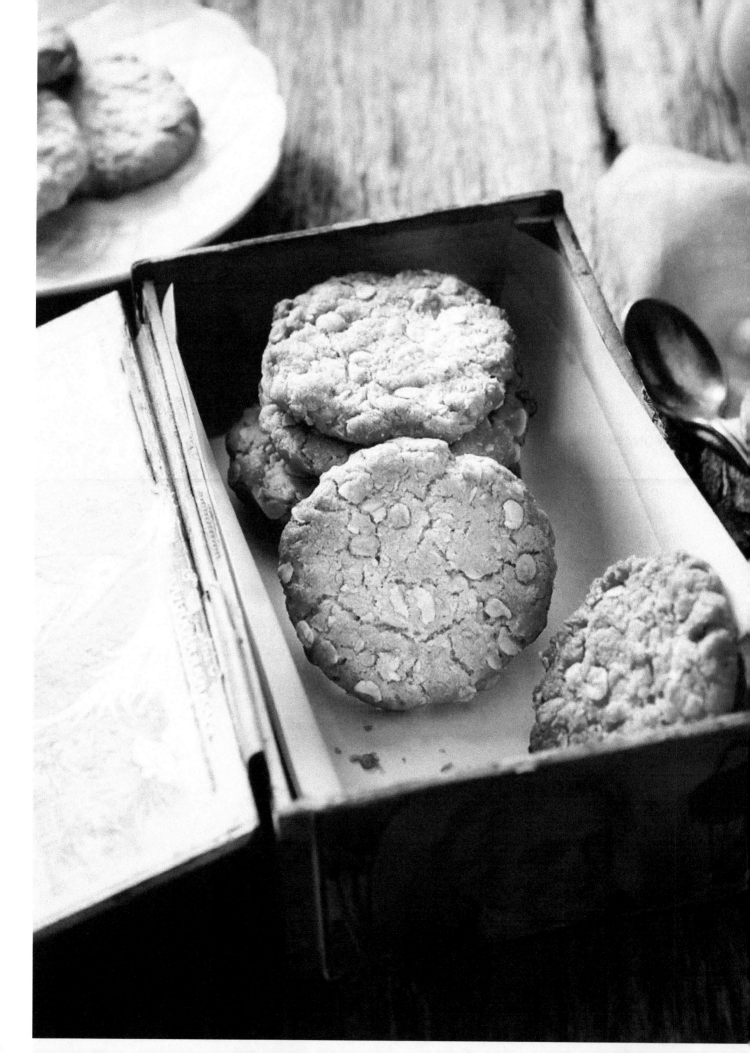

ANZAC
biscuits

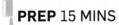 **PREP** 15 MINS **COOK** 12 MINS **MAKES** 18 BISCUITS

INGREDIENTS

125g (½ block) Fairy margarine

3 tbs golden syrup

½ tsp bicarb soda

2 tbs hot water

150g (1 cup) plain flour, sifted

110g (½ cup) caster sugar

90g (1 cup) desiccated coconut

90g (1 cup) rolled oats

METHOD

1. Pre-heat oven to 150°C. Line 2 baking trays with baking paper

2. Melt Fairy and golden syrup in a small saucepan over low heat. Add the bicarb soda mixed with water

3. Combine the dry ingredients in a large mixing bowl, pour melted Fairy mixture into the centre and mix together

4. Roll heaped tablespoons of the mixture and place on the prepared trays. Flatten the mix down with the palm of your hand until approx. 1cm

5. Bake for 10–12 minutes or until golden brown. Cool on a cooling rack

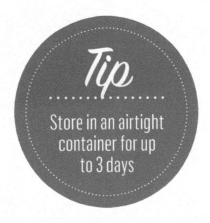

Tip

Store in an airtight container for up to 3 days

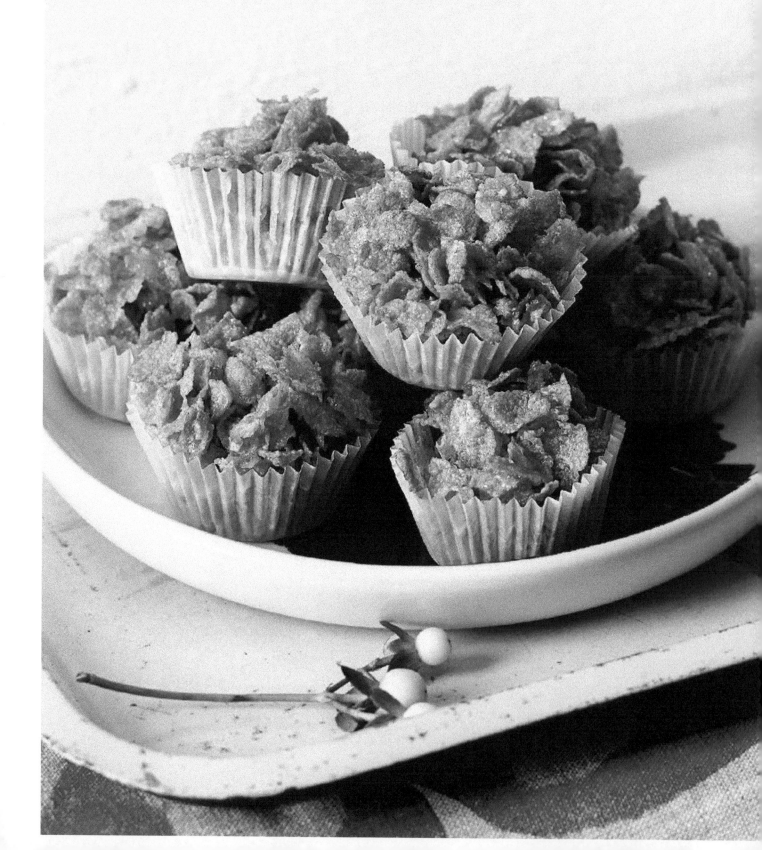

ADD SULTANAS,
DRIED CRANBERRIES OR
CHOCOLATE CHIPS FOR
EXTRA GOODNESS

HONEY *joys*

 PREP 8-10 MINS **COOK** 15 MINS **MAKES** 18 HONEY JOYS

INGREDIENTS

60g Copha

2 tbs honey

⅓ cup sugar

4 cups corn flakes

METHOD

1. Pre-heat oven 150°C
2. Melt together the Copha, honey and sugar in a saucepan over low heat, stirring until the sugar has dissolved. Allow mixture to cool slightly
3. Place the corn flakes into a large mixing bowl, then pour the Copha mixture over. Mix well to coat flakes
4. Spoon the honey joy mixture into muffin trays lined with paper cases
5. Bake the honey joys in the pre-heated oven at 150°C for 10 minutes
6. Remove tray from oven and cool on a wire rack. Honey joys will firm on cooling
7. When cool, store in an airtight tin

TIPS:

These honey joys are gluten free

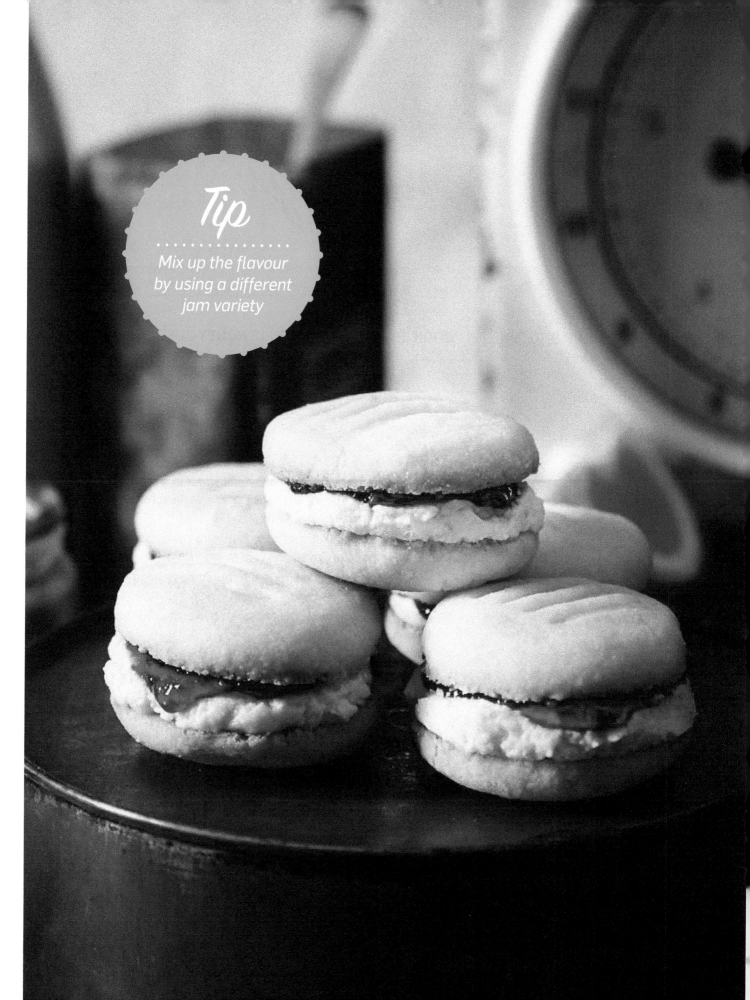

Tip
· · · · · · · · · · · · ·
Mix up the flavour
by using a different
jam variety

MELTING
moments

 PREP 20 MINS   **COOK** 12 MINS   **MAKES** 10 BISCUITS

INGREDIENTS

BISCUITS

125g (½ block) Fairy margarine, softened

75g (½ cup) icing sugar, sifted

½ tsp vanilla essence

100g (⅔ cup) plain flour, sifted

75g (½ cup) cornflour, sifted

ORANGE CREAM

60g (¼ block) Fairy margarine, softened

160g (1 cup) icing sugar, sifted

1 tsp grated orange rind

½ tbs orange juice

ASSEMBLY

Raspberry jam, to serve

Icing sugar, to dust

METHOD

BISCUITS

1. Preheat oven to 160°C. Line baking trays with baking paper
2. Cream Fairy, icing sugar and vanilla together until light and fluffy. Add flour and cornflour and mix well
3. Roll heaped teaspoons of mixture into balls and place on the prepared trays. Flatten with the back of a fork to make an indent
4. Bake in oven for 10-12 mins until golden

ORANGE CREAM

1. Beat Fairy until smooth. Gradually add icing sugar. Beat until light and creamy
2. Add the rind and juice, and beat until combined

ASSEMBLY

1. Sandwich 2 biscuits together with the orange filling and some raspberry jam
2. Dust with icing sugar

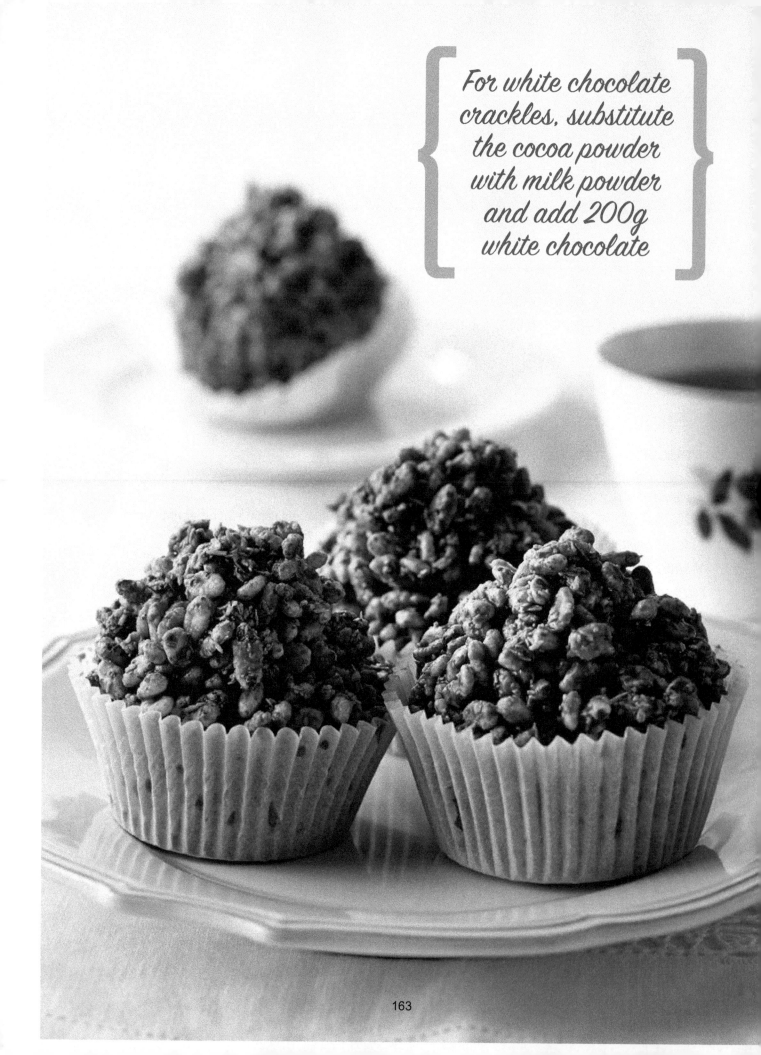

For white chocolate crackles, substitute the cocoa powder with milk powder and add 200g white chocolate

163

CHOCOLATE
crackles

 PREP 10 MINS (PLUS SETTING TIME)   **COOK** 5 MINS **MAKES** 12

INGREDIENTS

250g (1 block) Copha

125g (1 cup) icing sugar

60g (½ cup) cocoa powder

4 cups Rice Bubbles

100g (1 cup) desiccated coconut

METHOD

1. Line a standard 12 cup muffin tray with paper cases.
2. Melt Copha in microwave on high or in a saucepan until fully melted. Mix Rice Bubbles, icing sugar, cocoa powder and desiccated coconut in a large bowl. Add in the melted Copha, and stir to combine.
3. Spoon crackle mix evenly into the prepared muffin cups. Place in fridge for 1 hour to set.

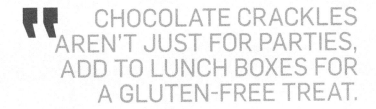

CHOCOLATE CRACKLES AREN'T JUST FOR PARTIES, ADD TO LUNCH BOXES FOR A GLUTEN-FREE TREAT.

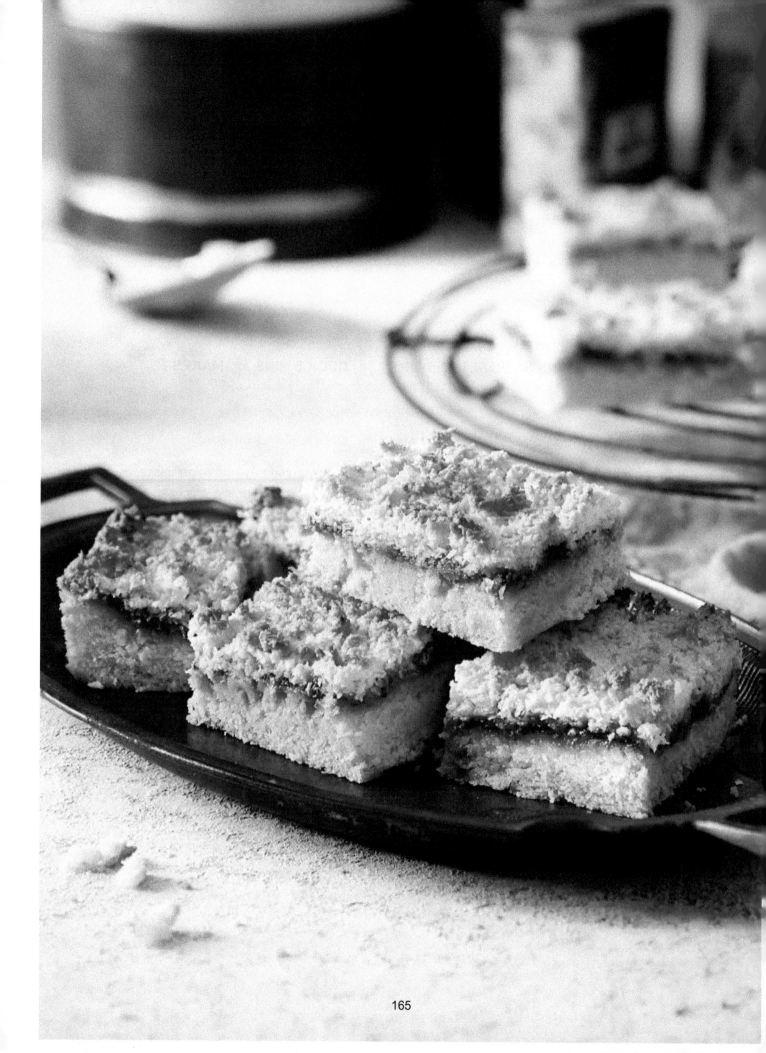

RASPBERRY
coconut slice

🔪 **PREP** 10 MINS   🍲 **COOK** 20 MINS   🧤 **MAKES** 12 SLICES

INGREDIENTS

BASE

125g (½ block) Fairy margarine, softened

110g (½ cup) caster sugar

1 egg

225g (1½cups) self-raising flour, sifted

TOPPING

90g (1 cup) desiccated coconut

110g (½ cup) caster sugar

1 egg

½ tsp vanilla essence

2 tbs raspberry jam

METHOD

BASE

1. Preheat oven to 180°C. Line a 20cm square sandwich tin with baking paper
2. Cream Fairy and sugar together until light and fluffy. Beat in the egg and fold into the flour
3. Press the mixture into prepared tin

TOPPING

1. Combine coconut, sugar, egg and vanilla together, mix well
2. Spread the raspberry jam over the base and spread the coconut mixture evenly over the top
3. Place into the oven and bake for 15-20 minutes or until golden brown
4. Cool in tin and cut into squares

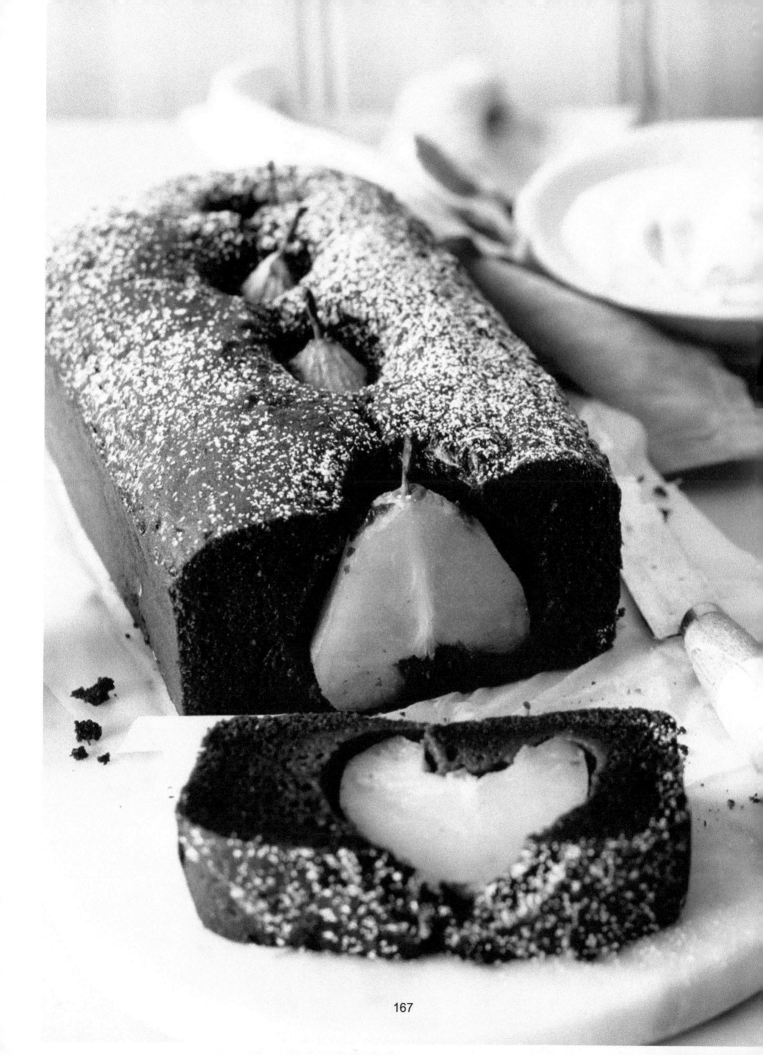

CHOCOLATE
pear loaf

 PREP 15 MINS　 **COOK** 1 HOUR　 **MAKES** 1

INGREDIENTS

540g Devil's Food cake mix

3 eggs

¾ cup water

⅓ cup vegetable oil

4 medium pears, core removed from base

2 tablespoons icing sugar

METHOD

1. Preheat oven to 180°C. Grease and line a 27cm x 11.5cm x 6.5cm deep (base measurement) (8 cup capacity) loaf pan with baking paper. Prepare cake mix as per packet instructions. Spoon one-third of cake batter into the base of prepared loaf pan. Stand pears in cake batter. Spoon remaining cake batter around and over pears until covered

2. Bake loaf for 50-60 minutes or until cooked through when tested in the centre with a skewer. Allow to stand for 10 minutes before transferring loaf to a wire rack to cool. Dust with icing sugar and serve

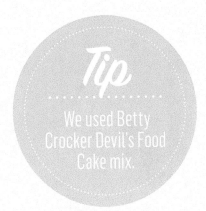

Tip

We used Betty Crocker Devil's Food Cake mix.

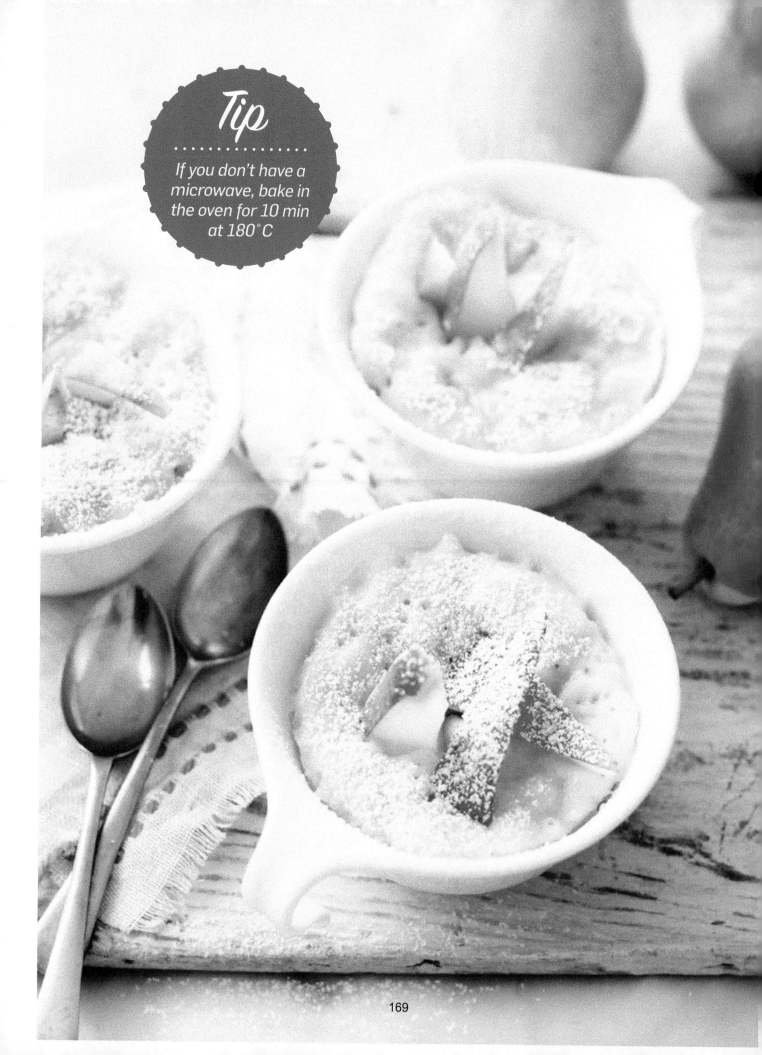

Tip

If you don't have a microwave, bake in the oven for 10 min at 180°C

PEAR AND ALMOND
mug cake

 PREP 10 MINS   **COOK** 1 MIN   **SERVES** 4

INGREDIENTS

1 large pear

⅔ cup self-raising flour

2 tablespoons almond meal

2 tablespoons caster sugar

2 eggs

⅓ cup milk

40g butter, melted and cooled

½ teaspoon vanilla

¼ cup maple syrup, to serve

Icing sugar, to dust

METHOD

1. Finely dice half the pear and cut remaining half into thin wedges. Combine flour, almond meal and sugar in a small bowl. Whisk egg, milk, butter and vanilla in a jug. Add to flour mixture and stir until combined. Stir through diced pear

2. Spoon cake batter into 4 x ¾ cup capacity cups. Microwave on high for 60-70 seconds or until cake has risen and top is just set. Stand pear wedges up in cooked cakes. Drizzle with maple syrup and dust with icing sugar. Serve immediately

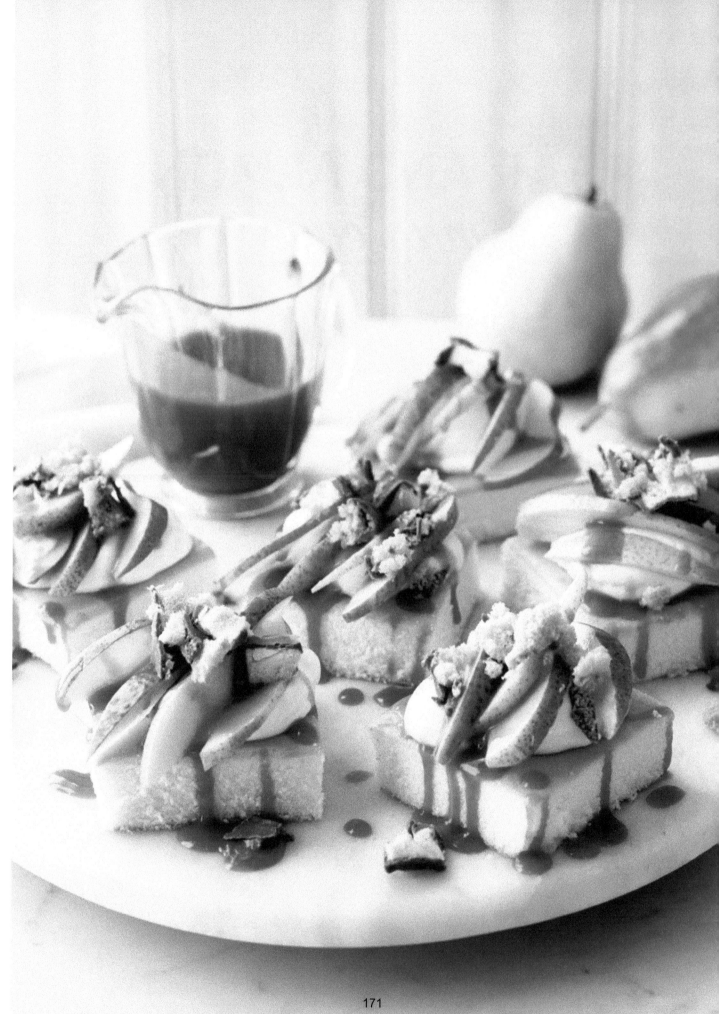

MINI SPONGE CAKES WITH PEARS AND
salted caramel sauce

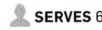 **PREP** 10 MINS   👤 **SERVES** 6

INGREDIENTS

*225g unfilled rectangular
sponge slab*

150ml tub double thick cream

*2 small pears, quartered, core
removed, cut into thin wedges*

*⅓ cup purchased salted caramel
flavoured topping*

*50g hokey pokey honeycomb bar,
finely chopped*

METHOD

1. Cut sponge slab into 6 squares or using a biscuit cutter, cut into 7cm rounds. Place sponge cake onto serving plates. Top with cream and pear wedges. Drizzle over caramel topping and sprinkle with hokey pokey. Serve

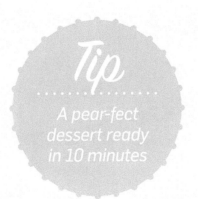

Tip

*A pear-fect
dessert ready
in 10 minutes*

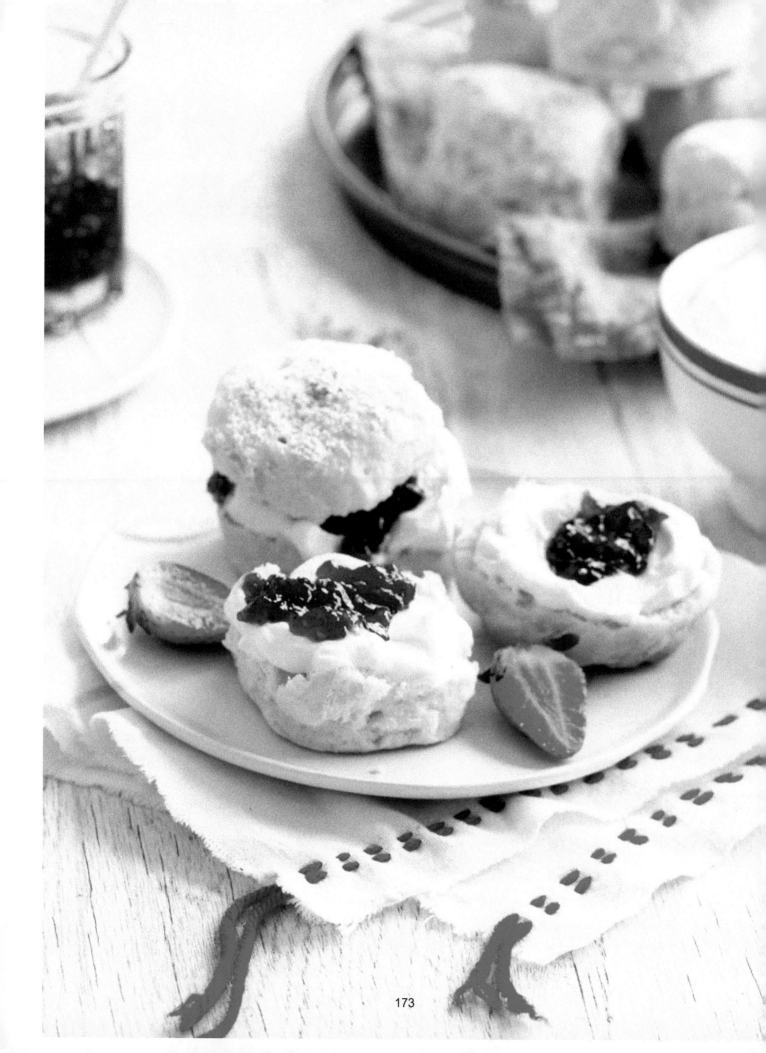

BUTTERMILK & VANILLA BEAN
scones

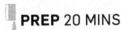 **PREP** 20 MINS **COOK** 20-23 MINS 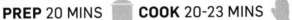 **MAKES** 12

INGREDIENTS

3 cups self-raising flour

2 teaspoons baking powder

½ teaspoon salt

¼ cup caster sugar

4 tablespoons (80 g) Western Star
Spreadable Original Soft, chilled

1½ cups buttermilk (plus extra
for brushing)

1 teaspoon vanilla bean paste
or extract

Icing sugar, for dusting

300 mL Western Star Thickened
Cream, whipped, and raspberry jam,
to serve

METHOD

1. Preheat oven to 220˚C/200˚C fan-forced. Place flour,
   baking powder, salt and sugar into a large bowl. Dot
   with the Western Star Spreadable Original Soft. Using
   your fingertips, rub together until mixture resembles
   fine breadcrumbs

2. Make a well in the centre of the dry ingredients. Whisk
   buttermilk and vanilla in a jug. Pour mixture into dry
   ingredients. Using a dinner knife, quickly mix until just
   combined (add a little more buttermilk to the mixture
   if needed). Pull dough together into a rough ball. Turn
   onto a lightly floured surface and gently knead just
   until a smooth dough forms. Press the dough into a
   3 cm thick circle. Using a 5 cm cookie cutter dusted
   with flour, cut 12 rounds from the dough (re-rolling
   dough as necessary)

3. Place scones close together onto a lightly greased
   baking tray lined with baking paper. Brush tops with
   extra buttermilk. Bake for 20-23 minutes until pale
   golden and cooked through. Remove scones from pan
   and wrap in a clean tea-towel. Set aside to cool slightly

4. Dust warm scones with icing sugar. Serve split scones
   topped with whipped cream and raspberry jam. Add
   fresh seasonal berries, if liked

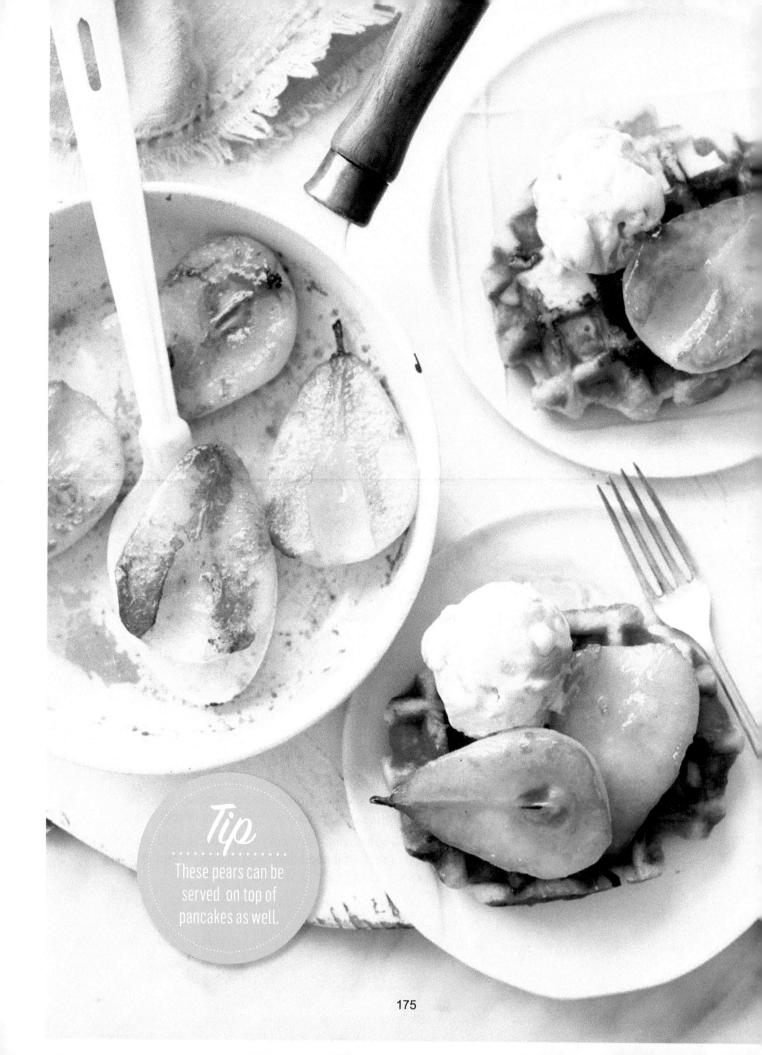

Tip

These pears can be
served on top of
pancakes as well.

WAFFLES WITH CARAMEL ICE CREAM
and pears

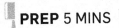 **PREP** 5 MINS **COOK** 10 MINS 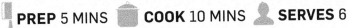 **SERVES** 6

INGREDIENTS

25g butter

2 tablespoon brown sugar

6 small pears, peeled, halved

6 thick waffles

Salted caramel ice cream, to serve

METHOD

1. Melt butter in a frying pan over medium heat. When sizzling add the brown sugar and stir until sugar has melted. Add pears, cut side down and cook for 3 minutes. Turn and cook for 3 minutes or until pears are caramelised and softened. Remove from heat and cool

2. Toast waffles and place onto serving plates. Top with a small scoop of ice cream. Place pear and sauce over ice cream and serve immediately

Lightning Source UK Ltd.
Milton Keynes UK
UKHW050652240521
384264UK00004B/42